THE
CANCER
KILLERS

THE CAUSE IS THE CURE

DR. CHARLES MAJORS

Cancer Killer

DR. BEN LERNER

New York Times Best-Selling Author

with **SAYER JI**

Founder of GreenMedInfo.com

ADDITIONAL AUTHORS:

Kimberly Roberto, Nutrition

Dr. B.J. Hardick, Nutrition
Co-authors of Maximized Living Nutrition Plans

Dr. Fred Roberto, Fitness
Co-creator of MaxT3

TABLE OF CONTENTS

FOREWORD

A Statement from Dr. Raymond Hilu of the Foundation for Alternative and Integrative Medicine in Malaga, Spain

After treating thousands of patients who were very sick with cancer, I can confidently say that what we need to focus on is not the cancer. Our focus must be on the provocateurs, the agents that are causing the body to get sick in the first place. These are the real culprits that build up in the body until you start to get cancer, which in the end is simply an alarming symptom of the accumulation of these agents.

I can treat the cancer, but if I do not stop the accumulation of these agents—the real causes of the sickness—the likelihood is that the patient will never fully recover, and often may die. That's why it's crucial to use the proper testing and the proper therapeutic tools with the right intention. You must literally be looking for the right thing. If you have only uncovered the cancer, you have not gone far enough. You must get to the roots of the disease. Once I have found the causes, which are different for each person, I'm able to set up a tailor-made treatment to stop these agents, reverse the buildup and help the patient back to health!

Combining the proper diagnostic and therapeutic tools with the right intention over the years has helped 85% of the cancer cases we have treated to go into remission. That's an astounding result, but our secret is simple. We are looking for the right thing—the cause of the cancer. Once we have found it using the right diagnostic tools, then we can prescribe an appropriate therapy that avoids the use of the more conventional, yet dangerous protocols used by traditional medicine, such as chemotherapy or radiation.

I consider a cancer tumor to be like a dangerous wildfire, and doctors have the obligation to extinguish it. This sounds very obvious and easy. So why is it, then, that in many cases these flames continue to burn unabated or are left smoldering, only to reappear later in full fury?

The answer is just as obvious: doctors are usually not removing the fuel that these flames are feeding off; they're not getting to the cause of the fire. If you don't clear the undergrowth or dead trees near a forest fire, hungry sparks will find their way to this food, consume it and blaze even more strongly. The same conditions can exist in conventional medicine. Doctors fail to clear the body of potential sources of fuel that keep the cancer growing and spreading.

This book is going to help identify these sources of fuel and offer ways that you and your doctor can eliminate them. This will help give you the upper hand in the battle against the spread of cancer.

ABOUT THE AUTHORS

Dr. Charles Majors and Dr. Ben Lerner are both leaders in a network of doctors who provide a health care delivery system called Maximized Living. The organization was co-founded by Dr. Lerner and Dr. Greg Loman and it's purpose is to help people avoid unnecessary suffering by changing the practice of health care.

At Maximized Living, doctors hope to amalgamate a fractured wellness model and create a standard for natural care. This goes far beyond scolding people for eating the wrong foods or getting fat because they watch too much television. What they provide is a complete system of living.

The Maximized Living Health Delivery System is Based on Five Essentials:

- **ESSENTIAL NO. 1** Maximized Mindset: Understanding the true principles of health and healing and creating a mindset for success.

- **ESSENTIAL NO. 2** Maximized Nerve Supply: Restoring and maintaining proper function of the central nervous system through spinal correction.

- **ESSENTIAL NO. 3** Maximized Quality Nutrition: Pursuing nutritional science that sustains well-being, disease prevention, and ideal weight.

- **ESSENTIAL NO. 4** Maximized Oxygen and Lean Muscle: Engaging in cutting-edge exercise programs that work to facilitate optimum fitness in minimal time.

- **ESSENTIAL NO. 5** Minimized Toxins: Supporting the body's own ability to permanently remove toxins from the cells.

Maximized Living has the only network of doctors in the world certified in these Five Essentials. The organization's practices are based largely on family wellness care and transformation health events in the community. The doctors practice in the United States, Canada, Puerto Rico, and in a clinic in Harare, Zimbabwe, located in Central Africa. They serve as the Wellness Advisory Council to four U.S. national sports team: USA Wrestling, USA Judo, USA Weightlifting, and the U.S. Paralympic Volleyball Team. Maximized Living also worked with the 2010 Major League Soccer Cup Champions, the Colorado Rapids, U.S. Martial Arts, and countless other teams and athletes, from the high school and college level to the professionals.

Instead of just looking at ways of treating cancer, the group's doctors examine the causes of cancer and ways to prevent it. Instead of only looking at one disease in this book, they're ultimately addressing all potential causes of diseases simultaneously. Their approach is unique as is the information in this book. This maximizes your chances of never getting cancer. For those who are already facing this disease, this holistic approach in many cases can be engaged to reverse it, as it did for Dr. Majors.

Many thanks to Sayer Ji, the founder of the world's largest, evidence-based, open source natural health resource called GreenMedInfo.com. He was instrumental in helping show how this information is more than just a theory, it's a science.

INTRODUCTION

YOU'RE A CANCER KILLER

Of all the world's enemies, few touch cancer. No natural disaster, common trauma, crime, or war claims anywhere near the number of lives this group of cells called cancer does year in and year out.

Whether you're working to avoid getting it or you have been diagnosed already and are working to beat it, this book is for and about you. We want you to be more than a survivor. We want you to do more than dutifully get your regular preventive exams and hope to at least catch it early. We want you to be actively working to overwhelm cancer cells before they take hold or eliminate them if they have gotten the upper hand. You were born to be a Cancer Killer and that's what we want you to be.

No revolution in science or great discovery will ever take the place of the internal human military defense system. Your body is on guard 24/7, defending your wellbeing and ensuring you thrive. The cure for cancer has been discovered, and it's inside of you! No other discovery will ever match it.

When your lifestyle is in alignment with good health and your body's defenses are on high alert, your internal atmosphere is too strong for any enemy to survive. When you're truly healthy, cancer doesn't have much of a chance to cross your borders. And if it does, it will rarely live.

You can never take, inject, or implant something that will create the kind of internal strength you need. While there are times and places for traditional care, nothing in medicine can take the place of being the natural born cancer-destroying machine you're supposed to be.

Whether or not your body will be prepared is up to you. We're very opposed to the idea that you're a victim genetically programmed for destruction. You have a say about whether or not you'll develop this illness, and if you do, whether or not you'll conquer it. It's up to you to take responsibility for your future. We can give you the knowledge to beat cancer, but in the end it will be up to you. Your willingness to put these plans into action will determine whether you're ready to be a Cancer Killer.

Almost all people have the potential to be Cancer Killers, including you. As you'll learn, there's really no such thing as a disease called "cancer." Instead, what we suffer from is a collection of stresses we impose on our body that causes the cells to mutate and adapt to a hostile environment. These get diagnosed as cancer cells. Those same stresses can also interfere with normal body functions and responses, nullifying your power over cancer. But you can eliminate the cause and remove the interference through what we'll show you in the pages to follow. You can restore your potential, and your license to kill cancer. The cure is in your hands.

PART I:
UNDERSTANDING CANCER

CHAPTER 1
LOSING THE WAR ON CANCER
Even if We're Winning Some of the Battles

On December 23, 1971, President Richard Nixon signed the National Cancer Act into law, and the nation began a war that still rages more than four decades later. "I hope in the years ahead we will look back on this action today as the most significant action taken during my administration," Nixon said as he signed the historic legislation.

The law unleashed an army of doctors and researchers, and more than $100 million in federal funds for an all-out effort to find a cure[1].

Commanding this army was the newly created National Cancer Institute, a research entity under the National Institutes of Health with autonomous power and special budgetary authority. Its strategy would be to develop research aimed at eliminating cancer by bombarding it with toxic drugs and radiation, and literally cutting it out using aggressive surgery techniques. It has allocated billions to evaluate different agents in search of a sure-fire cure. Alongside these efforts, the medical industry also pulled out all stops, spending hundreds of millions more to research and develop treatments and new drugs.

Yet, more than forty years later, while we might claim victory in some battles, cancer is still winning the war. Our failure is marked by the continued growth in the number of Americans newly diagnosed with some form of cancer annually. The American Cancer Society estimates that in 2012 that number will have reached 1.63 million, with 577,000 dying from it in the same year[2].

This disease remains the leading cause of death for children under fifteen, taking more victims than asthma, diabetes, cystic fibrosis and AIDS combined. Recent facts show that more than fifteen hundred people die from cancer each day, the equivalent of three fully loaded jumbo jets crashing and killing everyone on board on a daily basis, as Newsweek's Sharon Begley pointed out in a September 6, 2008 article.

The total annual number of deaths annually, almost six hundred thousand, is 50% higher than in 1971. Even adjusting these statistics for population growth, we've made only slim progress at staving off death from what is still the number two killer in the United States.

Fighting the Wrong War

During its 2012 Super Bowl broadcast, ESPN shared a story about New York Giants linebacker Mark Herzlich. Mark grew up as the classic local sports hero, winning all kinds of awards in high school and at Boston College, including being named the 2008

Atlantic Coast Conference (ACC) Defensive Player of the Year. Sadly, shortly after receiving that award, he was told he had Ewing's sarcoma, a rare form of bone cancer. Two of the ESPN commentators discussing the story were Stuart Scott and Merril Hoge, both of whom had also faced a cancer diagnosis.

Scott is forty-five as of this writing. Sometime in 2007, he underwent chemotherapy after doctors discovered a malignancy in his colon when they were performing an emergency appendectomy. He reportedly continues to receive chemotherapy and other related medical treatments in an ongoing battle against cancer.

In 2003, Hoge, known as "Hodgie" on ESPN's NFL Matchup, was diagnosed with stage II non-Hodgkin's lymphoma. Examining him in response to complaints of recurrent back pain, doctors found a two-to-three pound tumor, the size of a small football, behind his stomach and around his lower back.

As inspirational as these men are, you might think ESPN's story would have been about the failure to prevent cancer in America today. You'd expect there to have been an expression of frustration over the fact that, after all this time and money poured into treatment and research, three athletes—one fresh out of college—actually ended up fighting for their lives against the ravages of this still way too common disease.

Instead, the show perpetuated the ongoing, media-driven fiction that if we throw enough money at medical cancer research, we will find a cure: the same story we've heard from doctors, research foundations, and the "Pink" campaigns of the world for decades.

Stories like this one from ESPN, while inspirational and emotional, continue to mislead and to hold out false hope. The reality is that while we should all be very thankful that we win some of these battles, the current plan has come nowhere near winning the war.

Is our failure to lick cancer really just a matter of more time and money? Or are we fighting the wrong war to begin with?

The war we should be fighting would be one to educate people about how they can help their bodies fend off cancer (a job that their bodies were designed to perform, and would perform if it weren't for that fact that modern society has inundated us with chemicals, radiation, and unhealthy lifestyles). This war of proper education would lead people in the right direction and provide real and legitimate hope.

We need to fight cancer this way. We need to instruct people on how to boost their bodies' immune responses to kill cancer cells before they face a full-blown diagnosis. We need to show them how to aggressively address the hostile agents out there that are part of what brings on cancer. As obvious as this advice seems, the war on cancer has been almost exclusively an assault on the disease, rather than an enlightened campaign of prevention that clearly identifies things that cause cancer to develop.

That's a war we can win.

CHAPTER 2
A CANCER STORY
Dr. Charles Majors: I Have Cancer

Out of nowhere I began having severe headaches, and nothing would help but rest. Over months, the pounding pain and accompanying weakness would come and go. At first, I didn't think anything of my symptoms. I attributed them to working too hard.

I had almost never been sick before. In fact, I was the picture of good health with only 12% body fat. For the last ten years, I had followed a diet that was low in sugar, replete with green vegetables and fruit, and devoid of processed food. I exercised daily. I even visited a chiropractor weekly to remove any residual pressure on my spine from years of bodybuilding, bending over patients, and actively pursuing water sports.

But as I grew weaker, I became concerned. My wife begged me to seek help. By then my headaches had become much more regular, eventually recurring daily. They began to confine me to bed for as many as three days a week. The only thing that helped bring relief for a short period of time was a chiropractic adjustment. While I tried to eat healthy, exercise, and get adjustments for the past decade, those first thirty years of life with the three or four cans of cola a day, the other processed and chemical-laden foods, and spine trauma had likely caught up with me. Like a reformed smoker, I still might have some consequences to face.

After months of trying everything, the conclusion was that I had to have a magnetic resonance imaging (MRI) to see what else was going on. The doctors had told me they would get in touch within a few days. But the situation, as revealed by the MRI, turned out to be worse than they had anticipated. It was only hours later that the radiologist called. I had four immense tumors in my skull—two pressing down on my cerebellum and one behind each eye. They told me that I needed to go immediately to Northwestern Memorial Hospital, the medical center affiliated with the University's Feinberg School of Medicine and one of the best health facilities in the nation. It also happened to be in downtown Chicago, Illinois, forty-five minutes from my home.

My family and I were in a state of shock. While my wife got our three children ready for the drive into the city, I had to call my mother to break the news. She took it the way most mothers would: she jumped into her car and drove two hours to be by my side at the hospital. She would help take care of the children, all under the age of nine, who had to accompany us since there was no time to make provisions for them to stay home.

When we arrived at Northwestern, I was hustled into a bed in the intensive care unit. The doctors prepared to drill a small hole, about the size of a dime, into my head to drain the cerebrospinal fluid trapped in my brain by the expanding tumors. I remember thinking it sounded like workman cutting into granite as the doctors made the hole for the drainage tube. As the fluid began to seep out, I almost instantaneously began to feel better. That was the easy part. The next step was removing the tumors.

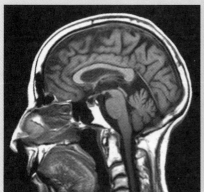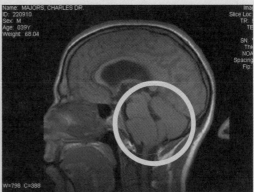

The MRI on the left is of a normal brain. The MRI on the right is of Dr Charles Majors' brain taken in September of 2010. If you compare the normal brain MRI to that of Dr. Majors, you can see that inside the highlighted circle are two huge cancerous tumors that are crushing his cerebellum, pons, medulla, and stopping the cerebral spinal fluid from flowing down his spinal cord.

My radiologist had referred me to one of the nation's top neurosurgeons who taught at Northwestern's medical school. I met with him the next day. Because of my age and where the tumors were located, he concluded that they were most likely benign and could be removed surgically. He never mentioned cancer, and the thought never crossed my mind.

Looking back, it should have. A series of tests had been ordered by the hospital before my surgery, and the results should have provided enough evidence to suspect a malignancy: I was severely anemic. My red blood cell count was so low that I had to be given a blood transfusion before the operation. There was also protein in my urine. There wasn't one normal reading in my entire blood work, but the doctors blamed the tumors and remained optimistic about my chances. Had they done one tumor marker test, they may have been more realistic about what they would find in surgery.

On September 14th, I had what was supposed to be a ten-hour surgery. However, after only a few hours, the doctor emerged into the waiting room. The news was not good. "As soon as I touched the first tumor, it bled all over," the surgeon told my co-author Dr. Ben Lerner and my family who were waiting for word. It wasn't until more than a year later that I was told the doctor also informed my wife and friends that because of the bleeding, there was a good chance I would not survive the night.

I still can't imagine what was going through my wife's mind at that moment. She and I had been talking about having another child, and now I'm sure she was wondering who would take care of the three children we already had. I was still blissfully ignorant, thinking I would awake, the tumors would be gone, and I could heal. Hours later, the doctors would tell me the news. Not only could they not take out the growths, my tumors were stage-four cancer that had metastasized from somewhere else in my body. I was thirty-nine years old, and the odds of making it into my forties looked bleak.

After surgery I couldn't eat without a feeding tube and couldn't speak because of the damage to my throat from the tube. I was facing a barrage of tests to figure out the original source of the malignancy. My doctors eventually concluded my organs were clear, and the source of the cancer must be my blood or bone marrow. A bone marrow scan confirmed their suspicions. Finally, a diagnosis! I was suffering from an advanced plasmacytoma, a form of multiple myeloma that had metastasized to my brain.

My grandmother was the only person in my family that I knew who had ever had cancer, and she died when I was in college. She was in her seventies, and I can't even tell you what kind of cancer she had. How could I now have cancer at such a young age?

In the hospital I decided to do my own research. I went to the Internet and plugged in multiple myeloma. Each search came up with the same result. There was no cure for what I had. I didn't tell my wife. I decided I wouldn't look anymore, but I couldn't sleep at night.

My mind kept returning to the words on the computer screen: "This cancer is incurable." I kept thinking that I would never see my two sons and daughter grow up. What would they be like? What would their lives look like? My youngest was only three years old at the time, and she would never really know who I was! How would my wife cope without me? I kept seeing my children with a new dad. The thoughts just kept going through my mind. I would leave a television on all the time so if I woke up, I had something to distract the brain where my cancer was expanding daily.

Finally, my surgeon and the head oncologist came to talk about my prospects and what choices lay ahead. It was a few days after the surgery and I was extremely weak. My wife and many of my colleagues from Maximized Living, including Dr.

Lerner and my close friend Dr. Marc Surprenant, were with me. To the Northwestern doctors, I had only one choice: It would be technology and me versus the cancer.

I was told the first attack against the cancer would be chemotherapy. A potent cocktail of poisons would be pumped into my body to kill off the malignant plasma cells . Radiation would be used to shrink the brain tumors. My cancer, but also my body, would be bombarded for days on end with drugs and radiation.

I would be nauseated all the time. I would lose my hair, I might lose sensation in my limbs. My whole body would endure the devastation wrought by the toxins that would end up killing both cancerous and healthy cells. And if I was lucky, after all this cutting and burning and poisoning, they said I might live another twelve months.

Another option, depending on how it all went, was a bone marrow transplant. "It's high-risk," the doctor told me. "But since you're so young, it's worth the risk."

At this point I had lost over forty pounds and could barely walk or even move. To go any distance, I needed a wheelchair. The neurosurgeons told me it was very possible I would never speak again, or eat without the feeding tube. How in the hell could my body handle another major surgery, poison, and being burned? I was almost dead already, and this protocol seemed likely to finish the job.

I needed another option. My body was broken, and I had to fix it if I had any hope of ridding myself of the cancer. I had to make myself healthy again, because I knew the cancer couldn't live in a healthy body. To do that, I had to eliminate the things that had caused my body to create the cancer.

People have asked me whether I was scared. I'll admit that, as the doctors and I struggled to understand what was wrong with me, I was. But by this point, I knew what I faced, and I was determined to beat it. To do that, I knew I needed to get to the root of the problem, the cause of my cancer. I needed a plan to help my body heal. I also knew I was not going to find the tools and guidance in this hospital, or through a conventional approach to cancer.

Fortunately Dr. Lerner, Dr. Surprenant, Dr. Greg Loman, and other colleagues from Maximized Living had already begun searching out alternatives, looking for a place where I could find the causes of my cancer. This was no easy mission. There is a crazy amount of information out there, and we had no clue what was right or wrong. Would a bad decision cost me my life? It's scary when your choices are, in fact, all life-and-death decisions. I was blessed because I had good friends, who just happened to be doctors, helping me.

After a frantic search, calling colleagues and reviewing research, my team came upon Dr. James Forsythe. He was an oncologist in Reno, Nevada, who had considerable success with the type of cancer I had.

The Northwestern doctors had been encouraging me to transfer to the cancer center affiliated with the hospital. Awaiting me there would be big-screen televisions and weeks of being pricked, poked, and blasted with radiation and pumped full of toxic chemicals. On September 23rd, I told them I had decided to pursue a different path, and I would be checking out that afternoon to head to Reno, Nevada. They wished me luck and warned me that traveling may be dangerous. I would have to take out the tube in my head, which would mean the fluids would begin building up again. They couldn't say what effect the air pressure from flying would have.

I was so very weak. My wife had to wheel me around in a wheelchair to get anywhere. I was so helpless and yet in a fight for my life. After leaving the hospital we only had hours before I had to head to the airport. I wanted to spend them with my children, who would have to stay behind. Although they didn't realize it, I was saying goodbye—just in case.

My wife and I headed for a plane to Reno. We were both so worried about flying because of the spinal fluid and tumors pushing down on my brain. At any moment, the vessels in my brain might start to hemorrhage. As dire as things were as we boarded the plane to Reno, I was convinced that I was headed in the right direction. I was on a new journey to discover and eliminate the causes of my cancer. The doctors at Northwestern were offering me man-made solutions to cancer, but it was time for me to seek out God's help. "God needs no help healing, just no interference," I kept saying to myself. All I had to do was to make it to Reno.

Dr. Ben Lerner's Story: My Friend Has Cancer

I've been through some difficult times. My father died on the front lawn of my family's home in Marietta, Georgia the night before we were going on a family vacation. I lived in Florida and had just got off the phone with my mother who, even though I was in my mid-twenties, was calling to remind me what to wear for the trip.

It was my first cruise, and she informed me that there was a night when the family would be dining with the captain, and I would need a suit. Fifteen minutes later I got a call from my eighteen-year-old brother, Rich, who said that he had just found my dad dead on the lawn. A year later my mother was permanently disabled from a stroke.

Those were tough times. Life has never been the same or, in many ways, as good. Yet with all of that pain, it paled in comparison to what my friend Chuck had to go through during his time in the critical care center at Northwestern Memorial Hospital, and the months that followed as he battled to recover.

He had a lot to lose and deserved none of what he was going through. He had every right to be angry and bitter. No one would have blamed him for losing hope. With what a malignant metastatic cancer patient has to go through in a hospital, you would have expected screaming, crying, and a deep, deep state of depression. Yet Chuck showed none of that.

While I'm sure there were many moments of despair, doubt, and agonizing pain, you wouldn't have known it by the way Chuck managed to remain supernaturally focused throughout the whole ordeal. He did it for all of us. His wife, his kids, his friends, and his colleagues, and for the purpose he knew he'd fulfill when he killed this thing.

Although he didn't and couldn't say much with all of the tubes and lines going in and out of his throat, his mental toughness was contagious and lifted all of us. His amazing wife Andrea, his mom Pat, Dr. Loman, Dr. Surprenant, visitors, and I were all moved to another level of strength and focus, making us push harder yet to find solutions.

From a health perspective, Chuck was a riches-to-rags-to-riches story. Before all of this, he was an ironman, putting in hours and hours each week seeing patients, consulting for other doctors, speaking in the community, and being a great husband and dad. Then, after only a short time in the hospital, he was wheelchair-bound and feeding from a tube. A few months later, he was at the top of his game again. He made his triumphal comeback by following the advice and care protocol we found for him and which he pursued tirelessly—the same exact advice and care you'll find here in this book.

Mostly, we hope you use this book, personally and for everyone you know, to do all you can to avoid putting yourself or those who love you through this kind of horrifying crisis.

CHAPTER 3
THE BUSINESS OF CANCER
The Sick Aren't Seeing the Profits

"It's difficult to get a man to understand something when his salary depends upon his not understanding it."   —*Upton Sinclair*

The pursuit of a cancer cure has meant big money for specialists in the field who research and develop drugs and other cancer therapies, and who design and conduct screenings for the disease. In 2010 Americans spent an estimated $125 billion to treat cancer. This expenditure is expected to climb to anywhere from $170 billion to $207 billion by 2020 as expensive new biotech medicines are introduced and included in treatment protocols.[3] Newer cancer drugs can cost as much as $25,000 per month, with a significant portion of that burden being funded out of pocket.

With this kind of money at stake, the line between the welfare of the world and corporate profits gets awfully blurry. There are many businesses that make their living off of this diagnosis, or even simply the fear of getting that diagnosis. The question should be whether the relentless and so far mostly futile pursuit of a cure, has as much to do with who's looking as what they're looking for. It also helps explain why an industry that wouldn't make money off of encouraging healthy lifestyles and natural therapies rarely chooses to investigate those propositions in the course of researching cancer cures.

The Screening Business: The Dark Side of Pink

The business of cancer produces strange bedfellows and inexplicable ironies. One of the original founders of October's National Breast Cancer Awareness Month was Zeneca Pharmaceutical, a subsidiary of Imperial Chemical Industries (ICI), which manufactured the blockbuster breast cancer drug, tamoxifen. Approved for use in 1977, tamoxifen has been classified as a carcinogen by the World Health Organization. ICI also produced millions of pounds of vinyl chloride annually, an ingredient in plastics that has been directly linked to breast cancer.[4] ICI spun off its pharmaceutical business in 1993 to form Zeneca Group PLC, which merged with Astra AB to form AstraZeneca in 1999.

The stated purpose of National breast cancer Awareness Month, which began in 1985 with the help of the American Cancer Society and Zeneca, was to promote the widespread adoption of X-ray mammography and annual screenings to prevent breast cancer. Its public relations campaign points to hereditary and dietary causes of the disease but neglects entirely the role of industrial pollutants, such as vinyl chloride[5].

"A decade-old, multimillion dollar deal between National breast cancer Awareness Month sponsors and Imperial Chemical Industries has produced reckless misinformation on breast cancer," Dr. Samuel S. Epstein, head of the Cancer Prevention Coalition and a Professor Emeritus of Environmental and Occupational Medicine at the University of Illinois School of Public Health, has said on his organization's website. "The ICI/NBCAM public relations campaign has kept information on avoidable causes of breast cancer from the public."[6]

All that aside, regular mammography, as proposed by National breast cancer Awareness Month, may actually prevent nothing and may in fact be harmful to women, based on recent research findings. Perhaps not surprisingly, the increase in this routine testing resulted in a soaring number of new breast cancer diagnoses and an inevitable boost in sales of Zeneca's products. What may be less easily explained is the fact that rates of more advanced, aggressive breast cancer have actually increased in certain populations[7],something that annual or semi-annual mammograms should discourage.

A recent study and editorial published in the New England Journal of Medicine indicated that X-ray mammography screening may "save" only one person for every twenty-five hundred screened. Among the twenty-five hundred screened, at least one thousand will have a false alarm, five hundred would undergo an unnecessary biopsy, and five or more would be treated for abnormal findings that would never become fatal.[8]

The health risks from these invasive surgeries should be a major concern because of the extra stress and even exposure to toxic medications associated with them. The U.S. Preventive Task Force, a federal advisory panel, suggested in 2009 that the risks of annual screenings may in fact exceed the benefits for women under fifty.[9] This elicited and outpouring of criticism from proponents of regular testing, including the American Cancer Society.[10]

Given these findings, X-ray mammography may be causing more harm than good in the millions of women who subject themselves to it annually, without knowledge of its true health risks. That conclusion is primarily based on the harms associated with over-diagnosis and over-treatment, and not the radiobiological dangers of the procedure itself. Here too, new findings suggest less is more when it comes to testing.

A growing body of research on the "low energy" X-ray used in breast screenings reveals them to be more carcinogenic than previously assumed. In March 2006, a paper published in the British Journal of Radiobiology, titled "Enhanced Biological Effectiveness of Low Energy X-rays and Implications for the UK Breast Screening Program," revealed that "recent radiobiological studies have provided compelling evidence that the low energy X-Rays as used in mammography are approximately four times, but possibly as much as six times, more effective in causing mutational damage than higher energy X-Rays." Given that current risks are usually based on the effect of high-energy Gamma Radiation, it's safe to say that the medical industry is underestimating the risk to women of annual screenings by at least that differential.

The Research Business

In the U.S. alone, the amount of money spent on cancer research is in the billions. The National Cancer Institute (NCI) had a 2010 budget of $5.1 billion and an additional $1.3 billion from the American Recovery and Reinvestment Act of 2009.[11] In addition, there are a multitude of societies and foundations that raise billions more, including the American Cancer Society, Susan G. Komen for the Cure, the Lance Armstrong Foundation, the Prostate Cancer Foundation, and the National Children's Cancer Society, to name a few.

Given this immense annual commitment to research, shouldn't we be radically farther along? More importantly, shouldn't the numbers of people diagnosed with cancer be dropping at some point, and shouldn't the cost of treating them be going down as well? Neither is the case. As mentioned previously, the National Cancer Institute has projected that costs of care for the disease will climb another $45 billion by 2020. Other experts have estimated that the costs are already well over 100 billion a year and will rise as much as $157 billion by 2020.[12] Doesn't this suggest that research dollars are not being used effectively or that we may be researching the wrong thing?

As a side note, another good question is: what would all of these organizations that are making millions to billions a year do if a cancer cure were found?

The Drug Business

Many questionable practices of the cancer industry have also popped up relative to the use of cancer-fighting drugs. As mentioned earlier, tamoxifen, for example, is a human carcinogen. So while it's a known cause of cancer, it's still being used as a first line treatment for certain types of breast cancer. Is it logical to employ a cure for breast cancer that ultimately may result in a case of endometrial or liver cancer?

There's no denying that fighting cancer is big business, and the cancer industry itself may be one of the highest hurdles to overcome before we can change our approach to cancer and find one that focuses on real prevention, and discourages the use of treatments that cause cancer.

Chemotherapy is an incredibly lucrative business for doctors, hospitals, and pharmaceutical companies. As Dr. Glen Warner, a Maryland oncologist, said recently, "The medical establishment ... [doesn't] want to see the chemotherapy industry go under because it's too lucrative. That's the number one obstacle to any progress in oncology."

There are certain forms of cancer that respond well to modern chemotherapy and radiation treatments, and there are those in the business of cancer who may cite things like improved five-year survival rates in order to justify their efforts. We're thankful when anyone wins their battle against cancer, but there are still far too many who don't win, and the death toll is still far too high not to question whether our methods are really more profitable than they are effective.

CHAPTER 4
CUT, POISON, BURN

"You cannot poison yourself into health. This is a LAW."
—Dr. Charles Majors

Conventional cancer treatments are the medical equivalent of fighting fire with fire. To kill a cancerous growth, medicine employs something equally hazardous. It bombards the patient with toxic chemicals and radiation, both of which might be considered lethal were they not being administered by medical professionals. The doctors hope that the cancer cells will be more susceptible to their potent wallop than the healthy cells. The reality, however, is that "collateral damage" from the treatments is inevitable. It's not a matter of if, but to what degree the damaging side effects will take their toll, as almost any patient of either treatment can readily attest.

The DNA damaging effects of chemotherapy and radiation are actual causes of cancer initiation and promotion. Therefore, the standard of care in cancer treatment today is also a cause of cancer.

The great challenge to using the chemotherapy and radiation approaches is that they're incapable of selectively harming the "bad" cells and leaving the "good" ones intact. As in real modern warfare, the decision to strike is often based on deciding how much collateral damage to civilian populations is deemed acceptable. How many healthy cells will have to die in order to blast the cancer?

Conventional Medicine's Main Approach to Cancer: Surgery

The first option among conventional cancer weapons is surgery. If a tumor has grown too big and it's blocking a vital organ, time is of the essence and you may need to remove it. But can the doctors ever get it all out? If they can, does it really eliminate the cause?

Cutting out the tumor addresses an immediate need, but it doesn't attempt to rid the body of what caused the tumor in the first place. Without that, what's to stop cancer from coming back, as it often does?

If you have faced or are facing a situation like this, the good news that you'll discover in this book is that there are ways to get to the bottom of the causes of cancer. While no person is ever truly cancer-free, we can make our bodies better cancer killers and increase our chances at preventing another diagnosis of cancer.

Chemotherapy

"As a chemist trained to interpret data, it is incomprehensible to me that physicians can ignore the clear evidence that chemotherapy does much, much more harm than good."

—Alan C Nixon, PhD, former president of the American Chemical Society

Many of the most commonly used forms of chemotherapy target the fastest replicating cells, tricking them into incorporating deadly chemicals into their DNA, or by otherwise blocking some key cog in the machinery of DNA replication. Take 5-Fluorouracil as an example.

The compound 5-fluorouracil has been used for forty years in cancer treatment. It tricks cells into incorporating fluoride-bound uracil into their RNA and DNA. This essentially poisons the cells to death. But it's not just cancer cells that are tricked. The effects are system-wide, and the chemical often destroys healthy tissue as rapidly as cancerous tissue. It's so toxic, that a dose weighing no more than three pennies would be acutely lethal to humans.

Chemotherapy involves toxic chemicals. If the chemicals used in chemotherapy spill or leak, the cleanup procedure is similar to any hazardous waste disposal: don't let it get on your skin and don't breathe it in. Why? Simply put, they're just too toxic. Yet now the doctor wants to take these same chemicals and inject them into your bloodstream. Yes, it may kill the cancer. But it's also likely to mow anything down—bad or good—that gets in its way.

Would it surprise you to learn that the idea for chemotherapy developed out of the use of mustard gas as a weapon during World War I? It began as an agent of death as scientists saw how well it worked on a body's fastest-growing cells. Cancer fits that description. Everyone knows that bleach kills bacteria, but would you drink it if you had a bacterial infection? No, you wouldn't, because you know it would kill everything else including you.

Knowing this, one wonders why any patient would consent to such a treatment, but when you're scared, you take the alternative that conventional medicine is offering. It's just not in reality the security people are hoping it's.

Does chemotherapy kill cancer? The answer is yes and no. Cancer cells are rapidly growing and weaker than a normal cell. The hope is that the chemotherapy will kill these cells off first, but everyone's cancer is different. That's why two patients with the same cancer given the same chemotherapy may have profoundly different outcomes. A person survives when the chemotherapy chosen just happens to work on that particular cancer in that particular body.

Dr. Ralph Moss is an author of eight books on cancer treatment, and a graduate of New York University (BA, 1965, Cum Laude, Phi Beta Kappa) and Stanford University (MA, 1973, PhD, 1974). Having reviewed thousands of studies as part of the research for his books, he hasn't found a single study showing that chemotherapy cures cancer or extends life to as significant a degree as the public probably believes. In 2004, the Journal of Clinical Oncology published a study about chemotherapy's success rates in Australia and the U.S. over a five-year period. It concluded that, when looking at how many cancer patients were still alive after five years, the overall contribution of chemotherapy was about 2.3 percent in Australia and 2.1 percent in the U.S.[13]

Chemotherapy is a dangerous assault on your body, and, after enduring it, your body must then overcome the damage from the chemo along with the cancer. According to Dr. Raymond Hilu, you must destroy the abnormal growth at a stem cell level to avoid a return of the cancer. This is another reason chemotherapy can be a complete failure at "curing" cancer because in order for it to reach the stem cell level the person would have to die. It's like throwing a grenade into a room full of rats. The animals will most likely die. But what's left of the room? And what happens if a few end up wounded and alive?

Radiation

Doesn't too much radiation cause cancer? That's a question you must ask yourself before you consent to radiation therapy. It's similar to chemotherapy when it comes to the side effects. It weakens your immune system and burns all the surrounding tissue so that the healing process is affected.

Radiation therapy is also known to induce secondary cancers by creating more mutated cells. For example, a woman whose breast is irradiated is more likely to develop lung cancer[14].

Cancer cells learn how to adapt to a toxic environment. When applying toxic doses of radiation and chemotherapy, these cells become better-trained and equipped storm troopers less likely to fall victim to the chemicals and radiation. Ultimately, radiation and chemotherapy may be responsible for driving a cancer into greater malignancy, at the very moment that these toxins are unintentionally attacking and weakening the rest of the body and compromising the immune system.

When the average pancreatic cancer patient, using standard chemotherapy and radiation protocols, lives no more than six months, should we say that the cancer killed him, or was it the treatments? Standard operating procedure is to write off the patient's death to an "exceptionally aggressive" form of cancer. Yet the cure may have transformed a relatively slow-growing tumor into a rapidly proliferating and invasive one.

IF YOU CHOOSE CHEMOTHERAPY AND/OR RADIATION, DO THIS

If you or a person you know chooses to take chemotherapy and/or radiation for whatever reason, you can still take measures to reduce the negative effects and increase your chances of surviving the treatments:

CHEMOSENSITIVITY TEST: First get a chemotherapy sensitivity test to determine which chemotherapy will actually kill your version of cancer. This is done with specialized Greek or German blood tests. These involve harvesting the cancer cells out of your blood, breaking them down genetically, and finding which markers are compatible with treatment of your cancer. It takes about two weeks, then you get a complete, detailed report that shows which chemotherapy or drugs are best for your particular cancer. This isn't typical of the approach in the U.S. where we don't look at an individual's cancer; we look at a category of cancer and see which drugs have worked best on this category in the past.

INSULIN POTENTIATION THERAPY (IPT): You may also want to consider doing targeted chemotherapy or insulin potentiation therapy (IPT). In this approach, the patient is injected first with insulin to lower their blood sugar levels. Cancer cells have lots of receptor sites for sugar. Cancer needs sugar to survive, and indeed cancer thrives on sugar. As soon as there is low sugar in the blood, cancer cells begin to starve. Because the cancer is starving and has to have sugar to survive, immediately the patient is injected with a small/fractionated amount of exact chemotherapy that matched their cancer. Because the cancer is starving, it eats up this chemotherapy, and the cancer has potential to be killed. This way the chemotherapy can be targeted toward the cancer cell; that's why it's also called targeted chemotherapy. Conventional medicine has spent years trying to figure out how to get the chemotherapy focused just on cancer cells so there is less damage to the rest of the body and now there is a way. The side effects are very minimal with IPT, and the patient rarely loses any hair at all.

Here is a website with more information on IPT therapy and a list of doctors who specialize in IPT: www.iptforcancer.com. Many of these doctors are very familiar with Greek and German blood testing as well.

PROTECT YOUR BODY FROM THE DAMAGING EFFECTS OF CHEMOTHERAPY AND RADIATION

There is an extensive body of experimental research that indicates a wide variety of natural substances — many of which are spices, foods, or vitamins — may reduce the adverse effects of these treatments, while simultaneously improving their efficacy. These natural compounds have demonstrated the ability to enhance both the destructiveness and targeting ability (known as selective cytotoxicity) of chemotherapy drugs to cancer cells, while simultaneously protecting healthy cells from their toxicity.

The following is a list of five compelling substances with both chemoprotective properties to help those who are who are undergoing or who have recently undergone chemotherapy treatments:

1. CURCUMIN: Found in the popular Indian spice turmeric. There are at least thirty-five studies indexed on the website (www.nlm.nih.gov) of the National Library of Medicine (NLM) on curcumin's ability to reduce chemotherapy-induced harm to the rest of the body. Another fifty-seven studies indicate that curcumin has chemosensitizing properties, enabling the drugs to work better at killing the cancer cells. Put these two facts together and you have what may be the most effective, evidence-based adjuvant to chemotherapy in existence.

2. RESVERATROL: Found in the skin of red grapes and other fruits. There are at least eight studies indexed on NLM on resveratrol's ability to reduce chemotherapy-induced harm. There are nineteen studies there on the chemosensitizing properties of resveratrol, making it another ideal adjuvant.

3. VITAMIN E: Found in wheat germ oil, mangoes, avocados and kiwifruit. Chemotherapy produces a huge amount of oxidative stress, which is why vitamin E reduces its adverse effects. You must make sure not to use the petrochemically derived forms known as DL-alpha tocopherol, as technically they may actually contribute to cancer. In fact, DL-alpha has been linked to increased pancreatic cancer mortality.

4. GINGER: Common spice used in cooking, and in teas and other beverages. Ginger is an ideal herb because it not only reduces chemotherapy-induced toxicity, but also the nausea associated with its use. There is also some indication that is a chemosensitizer.

5. SULFORAPHANE: Found in cruciferous vegetables such as broccoli, brussel sprouts or cabbages. This sulfur-rich phytocompound is especially effective at activating detoxification pathways in the liver, and is well known to prevent chemotherapy-induced liver damage. There are also at least six studies on its chemosensitizing properties indexed on NLM.

CHAPTER 5
WHY THERE IS REALLY NO SUCH THING AS CANCER!

This is a chapter that will no doubt create a lot of controversy and confusion. Right now you're thinking, "How can they say there's really no such thing as cancer when everyone knows that cancer is real?"

Knowing the Enemy

It wasn't until 1953 and the discovery of DNA that science began to develop modern theories of the causes of cancer. The dominant explanation, mutational theory, focuses on uncontrollable replication by rogue cells.

The behavior of these cells gone rogue is the result of multiple events destructive to their DNA code. Some inherited DNA sequences, or what are considered "bad genes," can provoke the mutations as can exposure to chemicals, radiation, and a host of other environmental stress factors.

Here researchers diverge in their ideas about the significance of these mutations. Some see the changes as cells just going berserk. However, a newer school of thought has recognized the alteration of DNA as actually coming from a natural adaptive response to stresses imposed on the body. And by seeing an intelligent pattern behind this activity, we may be better able to understand how to interrupt it.

Cancers are ridiculously smart. They adapt in remarkable ways so that they can survive in a body's internal, hostile environment: They're capable of building their own blood supply. They defend themselves by silencing cancer-suppressing genes. They activate tumor-promoting genes. And finally, they can alter their metabolism in order to acclimate to low-oxygen, high-sugar, and acidic conditions. Their diabolical self-protection system even allows them to remove their own surface-receptor proteins, to fly under the radar of white blood cells and avoid detection.

While random mutations no doubt play a major role in the initiation and promotion of cancer, it's hard to attribute these complex behaviors—exhibited by all cancer growths regardless of site—to haphazard changes in cellular DNA alone. It's become obvious to some researchers that much of the prevalence of this pernicious disease is largely a result of a normal, adaptive survival response by these cells to the toxic world both outside and inside our bodies that we expose them to.

If you look at the remarkable way cancers protect themselves, you can no longer view this problem solely as something pre-programmed into a defective gene. These cells are the result of your body adapting to survive. Your body is exposed to an increasingly toxic environment, an unnatural diet, and a loss of homeostasis. Of course, as these cells adapt (or mutate), they should be governed by the strict law of your immune system. However, as we continue to live in such a way as to compromise immune function, lawlessness prevails, and cancer thrives.

Cancer Is a Symptom and Not a Disease

What is becoming increasingly clear is that cancer is not a matter of genetically pre-programmed cells gone crazy, but a survival response—an attempt to endure whatever hell you're putting your body through. This trauma also rocks your immune system. So realistically, cancer isn't a "disease" but a symptom of the abuse the environment and you are heaping on your body.

Cancer can't overwhelm a well person. Cancer shows up when a person is sick! It's a symptom of an overwhelmed and poorly functioning body. Where mutations and adaptations are happening out of control and the body's defense system can no longer contain it. **CANCER IS A SYMPTOM, NOT A DISEASE!**

This is a hypercritical point: cancer doesn't make you sick. Instead, over time, your sickness creates cancer. In other words, you don't "cure" cancer by eliminating cancer growths. You cure cancer by getting a healthy body that stops cancer from growing and kills any excessive cancers cells that may show up.

The good news is that this removes the image of the cruel hand of fate deciding who will get cancer and who won't. This shows that the ability to avert the emergence of cancer, or kill it once it has appeared, is generally in human control. That said, modern society does not make the task of staying healthy and disease-free easy. Sickness in general, especially cancer, preys on the uninformed, and those that won't or can't act to defend themselves.

If you have this disease, it's your body's way of screaming, "It's time to change!" If you don't change, your body can't fend off the cancer, and no amount of treatment will make it right. If you don't have the disease, don't wait until you're sick with symptoms. You need to be killing cancer every day whether you've got a diagnosis or not.

Stop the Enemy in Its Tracks

Once we realize why the cells are mutating and why they need to adapt in order to survive, we can make the necessary changes to our lives. The priority for dealing with cancer is abundantly clear: we must halt the process to stop cancer from occurring, continuing, or recurring.

If you only try to cut, poison and burn without addressing why the cells are there, this symptom called cancer will likely continue or come back.

Sadly, the agents of cause are everywhere today. To stop this problem, you need to address a combination of lifestyle factors and do what you can to build a titanium immune system.

THE THREE REASONS WHY THERE IS REALLY NO SUCH THING AS CANCER!

TO RECAP -

CANCER IS NORMAL: Every body, even healthy bodies, produces thousands of cancer cells daily. Yet, not everyone is diagnosed with cancer because the body is supposed to manage and kill these cells.

CANCER IS AN ADAPTATION: Cancer involves mutations of normal, healthy cells that result in changes in a cell's DNA. While medical science has often seen these mutations as random gene expressions, there's a growing body of medical research that suggests that the mutations are not random, but follow survival patterns. The cells are changing their structures to survive against an external and internal environmental assault on the body. These cells are replicating as fast as they can and throwing up defense mechanisms to preserve their own existence.

CANCER IS A SYMPTOM AND NOT A DISEASE: The promising truth is that cancer can't flourish in a healthy body. Cancer shows up when a person is sick! Ultimately, cancer is a symptom, not a disease. It's a side effect that occurs when a body is not functioning and healing at a high level, and so allowing these bad cells to accumulate in abundance. If your immune functions and immune supporting systems are operating optimally, your body will deploy cancer-killing cells and chemicals at the right time, at the right place, and in the right amounts to destroy cancer and eliminate cancer-causing agents.

CHAPTER 6
ONE CAUSE: ONE CURE
Address the Cause, Remove the Interference

We're trying to show that, at its essence, cancer is a natural consequence of repeated exposure to stresses that we'll describe in the next sections of this book. The cells don't just mutate randomly per genetics. They're adapting to a poisoned environment as a survival mechanism. As a result, your immune system comes to a point at which it can no longer cope with these mutations, because the poisoned environment hasn't changed and is still forcing cells to mutate. To understand this immunity fact better, you need only look at the side effects from any of the drugs that reduce a body's immune function. One side effect is always a heightened risk of tumors developing.

If you view it that way, it's easy to see why the answer is not injecting more toxins into your body, which is already replete with them. Instead, solutions should involve detoxifying and taking out the stresses that are causing these mutations and adaptations. This in turn supports your body's own inherent defense system, and you're ready to be inducted into the legion of Cancer Killers.

The cancer industry has consistently stressed early detection as the best defense against cancer. But by the time a medical test can diagnose you with cancer, that cancer has already grown to at least hundreds of thousands, if not millions, of cells. That already puts your body at a disadvantage. As Dr. Otis Brawley, chief medical officer of the American Cancer Society, said, "One cancer cell is smarter than a thousand scientists." While earlier is better than later, by the time you've found several million cells through early detection, billions of dollars and a multitude of doctors and scientists don't stand much of a fighting chance against this insidious condition.

So if you don't have a diagnosis of cancer, you can't assume you're safe. Before that diagnosis, you've got to do something to become a Cancer Killer now! Where scientists fail, the power of your body can succeed.

Throughout the next chapters, we'll be addressing causes. Cause is the term to focus on. You may be used to the terminology like treat or remove when it comes to cancer. But we don't want you to wait to treat and remove, we want you to be pro-active and powerful, and eliminate the cause before you need the treatment. We want you to be a Cancer Killer.

When you address causes you remove interference. These causes not only effectively turn cells cancerous, but they diminish important organ functions. Your immune organs, detoxifying organs, oxygenating systems, and others are critical for keeping you healthy. These causes will interfere with the way these vital organs and systems work, and set you up for disease.

The Cause Is the Cure

There's really only one cause. It's called interference. Anything that interferes with normal cell life and healthy organ function can push you toward cancer.

So the cancer cure mantra should be: "Address the cause, remove the interference, and maximize function; Address the cause, remove the interference, and maximize potential, etc." This is a phenomenal principle for living in good health.

If we can target the stressors that cause cells to turn cancerous and subsequently interfere with the function of your immune system, you'll maximize your ability to fight. Attacking the cause is the cure.

Medical campaigns are often anti-cause. Susan G. Komen for the Cure published this statement: "A pooled analysis of the data from eight large cohort studies found increasing the intake of fruits and vegetables by about one serving a day did not lower the risk of breast cancer. And, findings showed women who ate the most fruits and vegetables did not have a lower risk of breast cancer compared to those who ate the least."[15]

Have we really come to the point where the commonsense consumption of fruits and vegetables in the prevention of disease can so matter-of-factly be called into question? Do we really need randomized, double-blind and placebo-controlled clinical trials to prove beyond a shadow of a doubt that our bodies can benefit from the phytonutrients and antioxidants in fruits and vegetables in the prevention of cancer?

"Cure" oriented campaigns generally only put prevention in the context of minimizing the causative connection between clear issues, such as smoking and lung cancer.

Sadly, breast cancer Awareness Month has not become a time of increasing awareness of the preventable causes of breast cancer but has instead become about simply early detection and then aggressive treatment.

On first account, a pharmaceutical "cure" is as unlikely as it's oxymoronic. Drugs do not cure disease any more than bullets cure war. At the end of the day, it's the body that is still responsible to treat and heal itself, even when an invasive approach is used.

This is not to say there is no value in early detection or aggressive medical care, particularly in the case of extreme emergencies. But if it were not for the body's truly miraculous self-healing abilities and the ceaseless self-correction process that occurs each and every moment within each and every cell, our bodies would perish within a matter of minutes.

The mystery is not that our bodies succumb to cancer; rather the mystery is that after years and even decades of chemical exposure and nutrient deprivation, our bodies somehow prevail against cancer as long as they do. This is a real testimony to the body's ability to hang on for years despite the abuse.

The primary causes of breast cancer and other cancers that will be covered over the next several chapters—such as neurological dysfunctions, nutritional deficiencies and obesity, exposure to environmental toxicity, inflammation, and estrogen dominance/hormonal imbalance—are entirely overlooked by this fixation on drug therapy and its would-be "magic bullets," and the completely dumbed down and pseudo-scientific concept that "genes cause disease."

With the billions of dollars raised and funneled into drug research over decades, the truth is that spending that time and money looking at causes would offer far more promise in the prevention and treatment of breast cancer or any kind of cancer. Addressing the cause and removing the interference would obviously prove a greater investment than all the exams and drugs on the market put together.

Changing Beliefs from Victim to Killer

Given the fixation on pharmaceuticals and radiation and the notion of having a screening alert you to your fate, it's no wonder that most people don't believe there's anything they can do about their lifestyle that would prevent and even reverse this disease. To illustrate, when polled, over 40% of women said they believe they will contract breast cancer sometime in their lives. This is well over three times the actual statistical number of women who will be diagnosed with breast cancer! But the prevalent fear makes sense when you realize that most women think all they can do is watch, wait, and pray. If you give them weapons, they might be more optimistic.

Yet there's an overwhelming amount of evidence showing the lifestyle-cancer link. Despite this glut of proof, a recent study by the American Institute for Cancer Research (AICR) revealed that nearly half of Americans believe there's almost nothing they can do proactively to avoid cancer. Whether this was denial or ignorance, the survey also showed that the "awareness" of a proven link between cancer and lifestyle was extremely low. The survey showed:

- 49% were aware that diets low in fruits and vegetables increase cancer risk.

- 46% cited obesity as a risk factor for cancer.

- 37% knew of alcohol's link to cancer.

- 36% were aware of the link between diets high in red meat (which you'll learn is commercial or processed red meat) and cancer.

While the public may be pessimistic, people do in fact have the ability to reduce exposure to carcinogens and other factors that might make them susceptible to cancer, according to a report called "Food, Nutrition, Physical Activity and the Prevention of Cancer: A Global Perspective" at www.dietandcancerreport.org. The report, by the AICR and the World Cancer Research Fund, took five years to complete and was based on more than seven thousand scientific studies. It is the most comprehensive review ever published of the science linking cancer risk to our environment and lifestyles.

An astonishing one-third of cancers worldwide could be wiped out through diet and exercise alone, according to the report. It also found convincing evidence linking excess weight, lack of physical activity, consumption of alcohol, and a diet devoid of plant foods to cancer.

The bottom line: unless we change our perception of what cancer really is and begin focusing more on not getting it, it will continue to ravage society and respond poorly to treatments. While some of its causes are better known—such as cigarettes, nuclear waste, or asbestos—others like stress, lack of sleep, a degenerating spine, or hormone dysfunction are more subtle and their cumulative impact on the immune system harder to gauge. They build up slowly and silently, until you get diagnosed.

Don't Say, "I Have Bad Genes."

Despite the increasing hype about the need for brutally expensive genetic testing, genetics really have little to do with cancer. As we already stated, random mutations and poor DNA don't explain cancer. It's also known that monogenic diseases, or diseases that result from errors in the nucleotide sequence of a single gene, are exceedingly rare. In fact, less than 2% of all diseases fall in this category.[16]

Following completion of the Human Genome Project in 2003, we learned that there are not even enough genes in the human body to account for the existence of all of our basic protein building blocks, much less explain the behavior of these proteins in health and disease states. From this, we must conclude that there are many other factors playing a role in the development of any cancer.

A 2002 article in the Journal of the National Cancer Institute summed up the danger of focusing exclusively on the risk from gene mutations and thus missing "opportunities to develop truly effective prevention strategies . . . based on a broad understanding of causative factors" (emphasis added).[17]

More powerful than genetics is epigenetics—literally above genetics. It's the science that reveals how your day-to-day choices influence your genes and therefore your wellbeing and the welfare of future generations.

Dr. Dean Ornish, a popular physician known for his work in preventing and overcoming disease through life choices, led research that tracked thirty men with low-risk prostate cancer who decided against traditional medical treatments like surgery and radiation. Instead, the men went through three months of comprehensive lifestyle changes in order to address causes. They altered their diets, established a consistent exercise regime, and applied stress management techniques for an hour each day. After three months, the men had changes in activity in about five hundred genes, including increasing the activity in forty-eight disease-preventing genes and turning off activity in 453 disease-promoting genes involved in prostate and breast cancers.[18]

Dr. Ornish, the founder and president of the nonprofit Preventive Medicine Research Institute in Sausalito, California, is Clinical Professor of Medicine at the University of California, San Francisco. Ornish received his medical training in internal medicine from the Baylor College of Medicine, Harvard Medical School, and the Massachusetts General Hospital. He received a BA in Humanities, graduating summa cum laude, from the University of Texas in Austin, where he gave the baccalaureate address.

The implications of this study are huge. Conventional wisdom often left people powerless to fight cancer: It's in your genes and there's nothing you can do to change your fate. This attitude turned the average person into a full-fledged victim. It also makes medical treatments the only viable option. Epigenetics puts the power to be well back in your hands.

As Dr. Ornish stated in the June 17, 2008 issue of the Proceedings of the National Academy of Sciences, "In just three months, I can change hundreds of my genes simply by changing how I eat and how I live … and it's not just limited to men with prostate cancer."

A November 2006 article in Discover Magazine, called "DNA Is not Destiny," further emphasizes these points: "Epigenetics is proving we have some responsibility for the integrity of our genome… Before, genes predetermined outcomes. Now everything we do—everything we eat or smoke—can affect our gene expression and that of future generations."

In 2006 Yale University researchers showed that genes played only a 25% role in determining the length of your life. Using that data alongside a British researcher's finding the same year that being overweight increased a woman's chances of developing all kinds of cancer by 60% shows that certain behaviors, such as being overweight, are far more significant than genetics.

"The genes have been there for thousands of years, but if cancer rates are changing in a lifetime, then that doesn't have much to do with genes," Michelle Holmes, a cancer expert at Harvard University, told USA Today in 2010.[19]

You can see how the genetic issue becomes almost irrelevant when exposure to Western lifestyles causes a rise in the incidence of certain types of cancers among ethnic groups or regions that have not had to deal with the disease previously. A clinic we started in Zimbabwe saw the consequences of the introduction of modern commercial living. While the area's biggest fear used to be infectious disease, we have witnessed firsthand how Westernization has produced a rise in the rates of heart disease and certain types of cancers, once rare to that part of the world.

The truth is that choices trump genetics. Your choices cause health or cause disease. So that which can cause cancer can, when reversed, be its cure.

PART II:
THE CURE FOR CANCER:
THE "DON'T GET IT" PLAN

The Five Cancer-Killing Essentials

Your personal fight against all disease is a lifetime battle. A battle you can win with the right battle plan. Yes, this means you do have to make some effort and get educated on the Cancer-killer lifestyle. With that effort, however, you have the power to stay well or get well. You have the power to be an overcomer, a conqueror, a natural born killer, and not end up just trying to survive.

*Remember: There's **ONE CAUSE!** That cause is anything that interferes with your body's ability to kill cancer and fight off any disease. There's **ONE CURE**: Remove the interference and maximize potential.*

So now you need to find out how. It's a tough world out there. You've heard people say, "Everything causes cancer!" You have to worry about foods, beverages, toxins, the environment, supplements, hormones, body function, and where, when, and how to exercise. It can seem so overwhelming and confusing that it's easy to just throw your hands up as many have and think it's too hard.

Do not despair! We've condensed what you need down to five basic areas, and created steps to follow that address the most common and likely causes of cancer. These are called the Five Cancer-killing Essentials. Your involvement in these Essentials can make your body a Cancer-killing Machine again once you embrace a cancer-killing lifestyle.

The next five chapters will dive deeper into each Essential, showing how each one plays a critical role in killing cancer and suggesting the steps to put them to work in your life. Your goal is to develop a cause-addressing lifestyle that's no longer a destructive force in your life, but rather a force to help your body protect itself now and in the future.

THE FIVE CANCER-KILLING ESSENTIALS

1. **MAXIMIZED MINDSET**

2. **MAXIMIZED NERVE SUPPLY**

3. **MAXIMIZED QUALITY NUTRITION**

4. **MAXIMIZED OXYGEN AND LEAN MUSCLE**

5. **MINIMIZED TOXINS**

A Life-and-Death Message on Lifestyle from Dr. Majors

Just because you think you eat right or "pretty good," think you get enough exercise, or even see a chiropractor regularly or occasionally, does not mean you're protected from cancer! Doing these things correctly prevents or fights cancer.

I was working out, eating well, and getting adjusted for years. If you looked at me, I looked healthy! But I wasn't. The cancers they found in my body had been building for a long time.

With nutrition, I was eating a lot of fitness foods without a focus on quality, and my supplements were mostly synthetic rather than whole foods.

I also didn't work out to support a healthy system, I just lifted heavy weights. So I looked great, but wasn't developing the kind of oxygen-efficient body that makes one the most effective Cancer Killer.

If you don't optimize and maintain your central nervous system, you're negating the area that plays the largest role in helping your immune system handle today's toxic environment.

I was getting adjusted every week, but the wrong way. It wasn't corrective care. After fourteen years of care, my cervical spine was still in terrible condition and continuing to interfere with nerve supply to organs and tissues.

On top of all that, I'd never addressed the massive toxic overload that my body was under. I'd lived in several new homes and office build outs the last several years before my diagnosis. Because of the new construction, I'd been exposed to all of the chemically-treated building materials that emit gas that's absorbed by the body but can't be metabolized without help.

So, yes, I appeared perfectly healthy! I looked like I ate healthy! I was adjusted, but it wasn't corrective care and it was done the wrong way. Additionally, the toxic burden I'd been exposed to was rapidly overwhelming my system.

That's why it's so important to never judge your health by the way you look physically, or because you think you do one area like nutrition or fitness pretty well. Your ability to be truly well and prevent chronic disease is determined by how closely you live according to these Five Essentials.

CHAPTER 7
CANCER-KILLING ESSENTIAL NO. 1: MAXIMIZED MINDSET

"The mind has great influence over the body, and maladies often have their origin there." — *Moliere*

The Killer Mindset

Understanding cancer and knowing the truth about your ability to fight and kill it's so critical to taking and committing to the right actions, that we made it the No. 1 Essential.

There's no doubt that if you believe you have no control over your health, you won't. On the other hand, if you believe you have the power to be or get well, you can become a powerful Cancer Killer. You have something to say about your future! You're not some machine pre-programmed genetically for success or failure, joy or depression, health or disease.

By making your internal atmosphere so strong through informed living, this enemy will flee the battlefield. Any that stay will be terminated. But in order to achieve this ability, you have to take responsibility. If you never want to find yourself in a hospital bed with tubes coming out of your arms, looking up at the ceiling and at God, then get control of your thinking right now when it comes to your lifestyle.

Don't say you don't have the discipline. We've seen too many people who get cancer suddenly become very disciplined and their mind very focused. They start to eat right, take supplements, exercise, make all their chiropractic appointments, get rest, de-stress, and spend the time with loved ones and friends they somehow never had the time to do before.

If you're reading this book because you never want to be told you have cancer, then read carefully the passages below that are written for people that do have cancer. You'll see the kind of mindset of control and responsibility you want to have now, so that you're not reading it later in order to overcome it.

So many people have put families, jobs, and other priorities in front of their own wellbeing. You're no good to God, your job, or your family if you're sick or dead! On an airliner, the flight attendant always tell you to put on your own oxygen mask before assisting others. That's because if you pass out, you can't help the other people counting on you. Take action and take responsibility, and do it immediately. This is the kind of Cancer-killer attitude we all need.

The Mind of the Overcomer: The Killer Instinct

As doctors and Cancer Killers can attest, attitude and the certainty in your body's ability to heal mean everything when facing this serious threat.

Dr. Bernie Siegel, leading oncologist, speaker, and author on the topic of beating cancer, noticed after years of watching patients live or die under his care that there was something unique about the attitude of those who overcame their sickness.

As Dr. Siegel pointed out, although given the same treatments for the same conditions, some died and some survived. He noted that the unique thread common to those who lived was that they had the powerful coping mindset of an overcomer. Overcomers do not feel like victims. They take action and know they will win!

In the ESPN piece we shared earlier, the athletes survived cancers that often take others out. You'll hear their overcoming mindset in what they had to say. Stuart Scott told ESPN, "I'm better. I'm stronger. You're not going to beat me." Merill Hoge also said he was ready to fight back. "It is destroyable; it is beatable. You have everything in you to do it. The mind is a powerful thing. There is no doubt, come May, I'll be cancer free; five years after that, I'll be cured. I'll be a better man. This has been a blessing."

And shortly after Mark Herzlich came off the plane to play in the 2012 Super Bowl in Indianapolis, Indiana, he tweeted, "Two years ago I was told I might never walk again. I just WALKED off a plane in Indy to play in the 46th Super Bowl. Take That Sh*t Cancer."

You need to be more than a survivor! Mentally, like these football players, you need to have a killer instinct to be a Cancer Killer. All things become possible as doubt, fear, and anxiety are expelled from your mind ... and body.

THINKING LIKE A CANCER KILLER IF YOU'VE BEEN DIAGNOSED
- BY DR. CHARLES MAJORS

STEP 1: First, you have to quit being a victim! You can't have the "poor me" mindset. If you're the victim, then you'll have a hard time gaining control of your mind, emotions, or decisions.

STEP 2: In order for you to get yourself under control, you have to take responsibility for your cancer. You created this. And as soon as you recognize that you caused the cancer, you also realize that it's within your power to reverse it.

STEP 3: Can you see your cancer as an opportunity rather than a tragedy? It's your choice how you want to see it. If you have the mindset that your cancer is a tragedy, then you'll approach it differently than if you see it as an opportunity to get closer to your family, make every day count, and find a real purpose in life.

STEP 4: You have to wake up every morning realizing, "It's possible!" Believe in the whole truth and not just the facts. The fact that you have a bad diagnosis or a positive test is not as powerful as the truth that you can overcome this circumstance and be healed. You face the facts, but you keep the faith, the faith of knowing that God needs no help healing. You have to wake up every morning saying to yourself, "If one person beat this cancer and got healthy, then I can do it too!"

Are you looking in the mirror and seeing a strong healthy person? Are you saying recovery is possible? Or are you fixating on your disease and remembering the doctors who told you there's no cure or your chances are only 50/50? Remember, those are facts—but they're not the whole truth.

A Healthy Brain: Build Peace, Don't Manage Stress

You don't do "poverty management," you do financial management or wealth accumulation. Similarly, don't manage stress. Instead, build peace.

In addition to the mindset of affirmative lifestyle, getting healthy thinking under control is an important part of Essential No. 1 as well. Constant stress and negative thinking suppress the body's immune system, alter digestive functions, and cause the continual production of negative stress hormones.

Most people are drip-feeding negative, toxic thoughts into their system all day from the time they wake up: the TV news, the newspaper, the radio news on the way to work, and then the news at night. If you look at the front page of most major papers, the world looks like it's going to end. So don't look at it or listen to it!

Read, listen, and get help from others in the area of positive thinking. Do your best to surround yourself with the positive. Don't write off stressful thoughts as normal for your situation. Be abnormal, be hopeful, and be optimistic.

You also need sleep. Your body heals when it's at rest, and sleep deprivation throws off important hormones and brain functions, and releases bad stress chemicals. The average person is at least 365 hours short of sleep each year. Americans are also sick—so be different and get some rest.

CHAPTER 8

CANCER-KILLING ESSENTIAL NO. 2: MAXIMIZED NERVE SUPPLY

The fact that your central nervous system (brain, spinal cord, and nerves) controls every cell, organ, and tissue in your body is a fact not nearly enough people consider. In reality, Essential No. 2, Maximum Nerve Supply, is vitally important, but often the most overlooked cause of interference to consider when searching for the cause of disease or attempting to assess a patient's health.

You have a connection between your nervous system and your body that works like this: All day long, the brain, spinal cord, and nerves carry chemical and physical messages to the body. Additionally, the body sends its physiological demands back to and through the central nervous system.

It's simple, yet infinitely complex. If this two-way communication back and forth between central nervous system and body goes on without interference, then the body is set up to function like it should. It's like having a good mobile phone connection; without it, your conversation may not be heard or understood. For this kind of intelligible back-and-forth communication to occur, the central nervous system must be protected from damage or interference by the skull and spinal column.

Although the spine and the skull are designed to provide protection, your spine and body are subject to a whole lot of physical, chemical, and emotional trauma in today's world that they were never intended to endure. As a result, it's common and likely for these bones to shift abnormally out of place and cause pressure on parts of the central nervous system.

When these bones move out of place, it's like the body is dealing with that bad cell phone connection, healthy communication breaks down, and messages don't get through. There is interference on the line. A displaced spine and skull end up interfering with the nerve-body pathways and so cause poor cell, organ, and tissue functions.

The longer this nerve interference exists, the more damage occurs to the central nervous system and the organs and tissues it supplies. This interference can limit a body's ability to produce normal cells, hinder critical detoxifying mechanisms, and badly compromise immune and other life-sustaining functions; all of which will threaten the body's ability to win its daily fight against cancer.

The Two Supersystems

The central nervous system and the immune system are the two supersystems of your body. The immune system involves areas of your body like the lymph nodes, thymus, spleen, and bone marrow—and the pathology-fighting elements they produce. These two supersystems manage the body's ability to adapt to the changing and too often hostile environment you live in.[20]

The central nervous system sends messages out to modulate immune functions, and also receives messages back from the immune system. If this cross-talk is maintained, you're in good shape. If this communication breaks down, one of these two supersystems doesn't receive accurate messages on the body's needs and the body is put at risk.

Immune substances produced by the body like interleukin, interferon, and T-helper cells are all driven by chemicals the central nervous system sends out when these elements of immunity are needed. These immune substances play a major role in fighting cancers.

For example, to call your Cancer-killing systems into high gear, your central nervous system will call on the release of interleukin-2 (IL-2), which in turn causes several things to happen:

- GROWTH: The growth of T-cells that attack specific disease-causing agents.

- ACTIVATE: The activation of T-cells and natural killer (NK) cells, a type of white blood cell that knocks off viruses.

- ENHANCE: Enhanced T-cell and NK-Cell function.

- DESTROY AND RECOVER: The stimulation of Lymphokine-Activated Killer (LAK) cells that destroy tumor cells and improve recovery of the immune system.

If something interferes with the conversation between the two supersystems, the immune substances like IL-2 and everything they in turn affect are now out of balance. As a result, the wall of immunity is breached, and you become vulnerable to illness and infection.

Establishing Maximum Nerve Supply

Clearly you need to have maximum nerve supply. What isn't quite as clear to everyone is how to achieve and maintain a healthy central nervous system. It starts with taking care of your spine. If the spine maintains its integrity, the brain-body connection can work without interference. Any time your spine is shifted out of place, it causes that integrity to be broken, and organs and cells immediately begin to suffer.

THE NERVOUS SYSTEM

Correct the Cause: Correcting the Spine and Central Nervous System

Care that realigns the spine, restores the curves, and makes sure the skull and pelvis are aligned is called corrective care. The reason for this type of care is like any other part of the Cancer-killer lifestyle: it corrects the cause, removes the interference, and maximizes function. Specifically here, get your two super systems fully communicating with each other to aid in maximizing immunity.

With spinal correction, as long as problems are caught in time, before too much damage is done, the nerve supply can be restored. Even "old" problems can be improved dramatically thanks to the incredible healing ability of your body.

When many people think of chiropractic care, they think of quick relief from back pain through manipulations and modalities like electric stimulation and ultrasound. On the contrary, corrective care is not for treating spinal pain alone. To actually restore normal spinal position and its proper relation to the skull and pelvis, there is required a series of specific adjustments along with a uniquely designed exercise program.

This is not short-term treatment. It's really about a whole new lifestyle. Once correction is established, some type of retainer or wellness care needs to take place on an ongoing basis to continue with maximum nerve supply.

You may never have heard about this from your medical doctor, or experienced it in the past with a chiropractor, but it's a well-studied scientific approach that has been proven over and over again through thousands of patients that experience this every day in offices around the world.

To correct a misaligned spine, you need a chiropractor specifically trained on the protocols to restore your spine and central nervous system. If you have less than maximum nerve supply, this is a necessary piece of any effort to establish or re-establish a beachhead of good health.

The Tools of Correction

A corrective care doctor will utilize the tools that have been created today to properly analyze your spine for misalignments that create nerve interference. This evaluation will show the doctor specifically what adjustments must be done to replace misaligned vertebra and restore spinal curves. It will also show the doctor the exercises that will help your particular condition.

Correction can be a very encouraging process for those who have been told they've got a permanent arthritic condition or terminal neurological defects. This type of care helps to actually restore disc height, reverse some of the bone loss caused by decay, and reverse what is often considered the normal aging process.

Depending on how long a spinal problem has existed and the degree of damage to the tissues, corrective care can take anywhere from weeks to years. Again, restoring and maintaining maximum nerve supply is not just about correction. It's a critical part of the cancer-killing lifestyle. Just as you should never stop drinking clean water, exercising, brushing your teeth, and eating cancer-fighting foods, at no time should you ever disregard your central nervous system.

Compelling Evidence on Spinal Care and the Immune Response

Researchers have known for a long time that there is a critical link between the body's central nervous system and the immune system. Chiropractic researchers have been aware of it since the 1918 Flu Epidemic, when it was found that the death rate of chiropractic patients was one fortieth that of non-chiropractic patients.

Remember interleukin-2? A 2010 study showed the direct response between an adjustment, and your cancer and infection fighting system. "Chiropractic adjustments temporarily influence interleukin-2-regulated biological responses following a single adjustment," the report showed. For example, the IL-2 biological response for activating LAK tumor-destroying and immune-boosting cells was triggered.[21]

One could assume from this work that ongoing spinal correction and spinal wellness care should help to establish more ideal IL-2 levels, LAK potency, and immune strength on a long-term basis.

A study by professor and researcher Patricia Brennan showed that when chiropractic adjustments were applied to the middle back, the response of white blood cells taken from blood collected fifteen minutes after care was significantly higher than blood collected fifteen minutes before, and thirty and forty-five minutes after. Her conclusion was that there was an "enhanced respiratory burst" following the chiropractic adjustment. This burst is needed for our immune cells to destroy unwanted foreign chemicals, invading viruses, and the wrong bacteria.

AIDS is essentially a disease of the immune system losing the war against a deadly virus. Researchers took a group of HIV-positive patients and gave them chiropractic adjustments over a six-month period. What they found was that patients who were adjusted had a 48% increase in the number CD4 cells, which are important immune system weapons, while those that didn't receive the adjustments experienced a 7.96% decline in the number of CD4 cells over the same period.[22]

In a study reported in the Journal of Orthopedic Surgery, researchers found a possible link between chronic nerve compression and vertebral deformity affecting the thoracic region, and chronic allergy problems and asthma. It was determined that the adrenal cortex functions of these allergy patients may be in chronic decline due to ongoing nerve compression. Patients receiving chiropractic care experienced a 70% to 88% improvement in their condition.[23]

CHAPTER 9
CANCER-KILLING ESSENTIAL NO. 3: MAXIMIZED QUALITY NUTRITION

Most people know that bad eating leads to weight gain. While this is true, the same type of diet that leads to added pounds also causes insulin insensitivity, hormone imbalance, thyroid dysfunction, poor bowel motility, toxicity, and cell inflammation, to list just the major complications. All of these factors in turn can directly or indirectly cause cells to malfunction and, as a result, lead to the mutations and lowered immune resistance we've been discussing.

Modern nutrition has led to a large percentage of American children, and the vast majority of adults, becoming overweight or obese. The problem is spreading around the world. The fat problem looms so large that on any given day weight loss can be the top news story or the subject of the number one book on the New York Times Best Seller list.

Most ideas about nutrition found in pop culture focus on looking good in a swimsuit for summer or a dress at the upcoming wedding or reunion. Yet the issue here isn't simply one of whether you look good in a mirror or fit into the same clothes you did fifteen years ago. This is much more than a question of vanity. Being overweight puts your body at high risk for an array of chronic diseases, especially cancer.

In addition to making you fatter, today's commercial diets contain endless toxins and lack the nutrients, fiber, antioxidants, and many other critical ingredients, that you need in order to grow healthy cells and manage your environment.

Testing positive for high triglycerides, high cholesterol, high blood pressure, high blood sugar, inappropriate levels of important hormones like insulin and leptin, and elevated inflammatory proteins are all side effects of typical American diets, and are signs of a body headed toward serious disease.

The key culprits we'll focus on in your fight against cancer: sugar, bad fats, and refined, chemical-laden products.

Hormones

Hormones are chemical messengers that affect virtually all bodily functions. Their levels and responses are profoundly influenced by all Five Essentials! In the area of nutrition, these hormones have a lot to do with body fat levels. Body fat has a big impact on cancer. Breast cancer, for example, absolutely loves fat-cells.

Insulin, also known as the "fat hormone," is a specialized hormone for regulating blood sugar levels and is involved in managing fats and proteins going into your cells. A diet high in grains and sugars, opposite to the one we'll be teaching here, will cause an excessive insulin response and ultimately lead to insulin resistance.

Insulin resistance is a condition in which your cells have become desensitized to insulin. This is the norm in overweight people. It forces your body to produce more insulin to have the same effect. Insulin resistance leads to a cascade of other hormonal issues tied to weight gain and burning fat, and can ultimately lead to full blown adult-onset diabetes. This disease isn't for adults only. It's becoming more and more common in kids, thanks to the Standard American Diet. (It's very S.A.D.)

The Key Cancer Factors and Nutrition

When eliminating nutritionally linked causes of cancer, we look closely at foods that affect the production of hormones and insulin, as well as issues such as weight, bowel motility, toxicity, and inflammation. We also address nutrients needed to support health. In doing this, we look at the three macro-nutrients—fats, proteins, and carbohydrates—when we determine what to eat and what not to eat.

Fats

The number one missing ingredient in the standard American diet is not a vitamin or mineral. It's the lack of intake of "good" fat. Surprising? It's not that we aren't eating fat; in fact we're eating way too much fat. It's just the wrong kind, such as hydrogenated and partially hydrogenated oils, trans-fats, and rancid vegetable oils. These are in most packaged foods. Where good fats are essential to hormone production, cancer prevention, regulating metabolism, burning fat, brain development, weight loss, cellular healing and anti-inflammation, bad fats have the opposite effect on all these functions, inhibiting ones we need and producing an oversupply in others. They cause problems in your cells and are related to cancer, heart disease, and neurotoxicity. They're also linked to much of the chronic inflammation from which people suffer today.

THE BAD FATS:			
Hydrogenated and Partially Hydrogenated Oils	Rancid Oils (Corn Oil, Vegetable Oil, Canola Oil, Cottonseed Oil, Soybean Oil, Safflower Oil, and Sunflower Oil)	Trans fats (Margarine, Synthetic Butters, and Shortening)	Pasteurized and Homogenized Dairy Products

THE GOOD FATS:
RAW NUTS AND SEEDS: Almonds, cashews, flaxseeds, hemp seeds, pecans, pine nuts, macadamia, sesame seeds, sunflower seeds, walnut, and raw nut and seed butters such as almond butter, macadamia butter, and raw tahini.
Olives, avocado, and coconut products including coconut milk, coconut oil, coconut butter, coconut flakes, and coconut flour.
ANIMAL PROTEINS WITH GOOD FATS: Grass-fed meat; cold-water fish such as salmon, mahi-mahi, mackerel, halibut, sardines and anchovies; and cage-free and free-range chickens that are hormone/antibiotic free and fed no animal by-products.
FULL-FAT DAIRY PRODUCTS: Full-fat raw milk, full-fat plain yogurt, butter (preferably raw), ghee (clarified butter), cream, raw cheeses, and kefir. Avoid commercial dairy products altogether and be cautious of allergies to them. Use full-fat, organic diary at a bare minimum. Non-homogenized is even better. Non-pasteurized (raw) is best, if available. Dairy products with reduced fat contain a higher percentage of sugar.
HEATABLE OILS: Coconut oil (best for high heat) and olive oil (medium heat only; do not let it smoke).
GOOD OILS YOU SHOULD NOT HEAT: Walnut, flaxseed, avocado, cod liver oil, hemp seed oil. These fats are good as they have the right ratio of fatty acids, but break down to bad fats when heated.

Proteins

Protein provides the building blocks for hormones and neurotransmitters. It's essential that you get an optimal amount of clean, lean protein at each meal.

Countless studies link commercial produced meats with cancer and heart disease. In contrast, naturally raised meats provide nutrients, good fatty acid ratios, and amino acids that are essential for good health. Many cultures have survived on naturally raised meats in the proportions that people eat in North America, without experiencing cancer or heart disease.

Animal proteins must be organic since, in the case of animals, you are not only what you eat, you are also what the meat eats. Toxins accumulate in high concentrations in the fats present in meat and dairy products.

When red-meat animals that would naturally eat grass are unnaturally fed grain, their fatty acid ratios are altered and their good saturated fats quickly become bad fats. As a result of the way commercially raised animals are fed and treated, they become susceptible to sickness and require high levels of antibiotics.

Grass-fed and free-range meats provide many of the fatty acids that are missing in the standard American diet. These are arachidonic acid, conjugated linoleic acid, and the proper ratio of omega-6 to omega-3 fatty acids, which your body actually needs for healthy cell function, to burn fat, to detoxify, and to prevent heart disease and cancer.

To see how bad commercial animal products have gotten, read some of the milk labels. Many now state: "The FDA has determined that there is no significant difference between milk from artificial growth hormone treated cows and non-treated cows." Clearly, milk from cows treated with steroids that accelerate production would change the composition of the milk and contain something you don't want in your body.

Many milk producers utilize recombinant bovine growth hormone (RBGH) to artificially increase milk production in cows. This process was deemed potentially hazardous and not permitted in the European Union, Canada, and some other countries. Milk from these hormone-treated cows has been found to induce a marked and sustained increase in levels of insulin-like growth factor-1, or IGF-1. Elevated IGF-1 levels have been linked to the progression of many childhood cancers and to the growth of tumors in breast cancer, small cell lung cancer, melanoma, and cancers of the pancreas and prostate.[24]

Avoiding this is difficult because the FDA will not allow companies to put "hormone free" on labels and most dairy companies co-mingle rBGH and non-rBGH milk so nearly all commercial milk, dairy, and infant formula products are contaminated. To find a list of organic and rBGH-free dairies in the U.S. consult the Organic Consumers Association (OCA) website at www.organicconsumers.org.

GOOD PROTEINS:
GRASS-FED, ORGANIC MEAT: Contains good fats in the ideal ratio for consumption. Choose grass-fed, free-range, and hormone-free animal sources.
FISH: Cold-water fish such as salmon, mahi-mahi, mackerel and halibut, from the cleanest waters (Pacific and Alaskan Oceans), and those fish that are lowest on the food chain, such as sardines and anchovies. No farm-raised fish because of their improper diet.
EGGS: From hens that are cage-free, free-range, organic, hormone-free, antibiotic-free, and fed no animal by-products.
POULTRY: Naturally raised, free-range, hormone-free, antibiotic-free poultry.
GRASS-FED, ORGANIC WHEY PROTEIN: Whey is the watery part of milk that separates from the curd. Unprocessed, grass-fed whey is a fantastic source of protein. It's bio-available, raises the master antioxidant glutathione, and helps to bind and pull heavy metals out of the body. Be careful: hydrolyzed and heat-processed whey proteins, which make up the majority of whey protein supplements on the market, do not contain the same benefits. Because their amino acids have been denatured through heat processing, they become virtually useless and potentially toxic to the body.
RAW NUTS AND SEEDS: Almonds, cashews, flaxseed, hemp seeds, pecans, pine nuts, macadamia, sesame seeds, sunflower seeds, walnuts, and others. These are an excellent source of protein and substitute for meat products. For best results, soak the nuts/seeds overnight in filtered water. Then drain, dry, and store in glass jars in the refrigerator. This releases the natural enzymes and makes them easier to digest and assimilate. Also, fermented soy products: miso, tempeh, and tamari.
DAIRY PRODUCTS: In most cases, these are best to avoid altogether unless you have the right, unprocessed product and no allergies to milk. If you find the right source, full fat raw milk, full fat plain yogurt, raw cheeses, kefir, and whey protein are good products.

PROTEIN TIP:

Have some protein with every meal, and most importantly, when your body needs it most (toward the end of the day and thirty to forty-five minutes after exercise).

BAD PROTEINS TO ELIMINATE FROM THE CORE PLAN:
Pork (highly acidic and large toxic load)
Conventionally raised poultry (chicken, turkey)
Farm-raised fish (these fish are fed and raised unnaturally so no longer healthy)
Shellfish (highly acidic and large toxic load) and large ocean fish (tuna, cod)
Processed soy products (tofu, soy nuts, soy milk, soy formula)
Commercial whey protein (if hydrolyzed, treated with heat, and/or from pasteurized dairy)
Limit roasted nuts and seeds (highly acidic, loss of nutrients, heat turns natural oils rancid)

Sugars: The Fuel for Cancer!

If an oncologist or anyone tells a cancer patient that it doesn't matter if they eat sugar, that person is just flat-out wrong. Like all causes of cancer, sugar interferes with normal, healthy, balanced physiology. What makes sugar even more of a problem is that cancer really thrives on it.

When a patient goes in for a positron emission tomography (PET) scan to see if cancer is spreading, what are they given? The answer is dextrose, which is a form of sugar. Why? Because cancer cells have more receptor sites for sugar than for anything else. The reality: sugar is the fuel for cancer.

Shortly before a PET scan is performed, the patient is injected with sugar containing a radioactive dye. The cancer cells eat the sugar, and the dye lights up like a Christmas tree when scanned. That lets the doctors verify whether the cancer has spread. Cancer cells, which grow quickly, are more likely than normal cells to take up larger amounts of the sugar.

In Germany on June 30, 1966 Dr. Otto Warburg delivered a lecture to Nobel Laureates titled, "The Prime Cause and Prevention of Cancer," which discussed the role of sugar in the spread of cancer. "Cancer, above all other disease, has countless secondary causes, but even for cancer, there is only one prime cause," Warburg told the lecture. "The prime cause of cancer is the replacement of the respiration of oxygen in normal body cells by fermentation of sugar (anaerobic respiration)."

All normal body cells need oxygen to survive. However, cancer cells are not like normal, healthy cells. Cancer cells meet their energy needs through fermentation. In other words, glucose (sugar) helps cancer cells survive and thrive.

High blood sugar and insulin levels also lead to elevated levels of insulin-like growth factor-1 (IGF-1). As mentioned previously concerning milk cows injected with hormones, elevated IGF-1 plays a major role in the progression of many childhood cancers and in the growth of tumors in breast cancer, small cell lung cancer, melanoma, and cancers of the pancreas and prostate, according to researchers at the National Institutes of Health. This has been confirmed many times.[25][26][27][28]

Whether it's the insulin, the body fat, the inflammation, or the hormones, many studies support the flat-out fact that sugar equals cancer. The Journal of the National Cancer Institute in 2004 showed that women who ate the highest glycemic (or sugary) foods were three times more likely to develop colon cancer.[29]

Do you ever see high fructose corn syrup on your food labels? This is even worse than regular cane sugar. Researchers at the University of California, Los Angeles, found that pancreatic tumor cells use fructose to divide and proliferate. The study, published in the journal Cancer Research, noted that tumor cells thrive on sugar, but they specifically used fructose to proliferate. And finally, it suggested that people who "reduce fructose intake … may disrupt cancer growth."[30]

With all of this documented research on sugar and cancer, over the past fifty years, how much of the money raised for cancer research has gone toward reducing the amount of sugar people are eating? Answer: too little to register.

Sugar Alternatives: The Good, the Bad, and the Out-of-the-Question

Sugar and its close cousins—corn syrup, high fructose corn syrup, fructose, and agave—are "anti-nutrients." All cause spikes in blood sugar. They include only an insignificant amount of vitamins and minerals and actually rob your body of stored precious nutrients. The natural herb stevia is the preferred alternative sweetener. Xylitol® is an acceptable alternate. These are both great ingredients for desserts and ways to satisfy a sweet tooth.

While alternatives like honey and Maple Syrup are natural, they will still spike blood sugar. If eaten at all, it must be only in raw, organic forms. And even then you've got to get some exercise regularly to burn these calories.

Chemical alternatives in the pink, blue, and yellow packages are simply out of the question! Saccharine, Nutrasweet®, and Splenda® are concentrated chemicals made in a lab and don't belong in any level in a body wishing to steer clear of disease. (See more toward the end of this chapter in "The Cancer Culprits.")

This disease-causer is everywhere. According to published reports, the top source of sugar for the vast majority of North Americans is soft drinks. Other sources include processed meats, pizza, sauces, breads, soups, crackers, fruit drinks, canned foods, yogurt, ketchup, and mayonnaise. Read the ingredients! You'll be shocked. This deadly white powder is consumed at an average of 120 pounds per person each year.

The Dangers in Grain

Grains, particularly refined grains, convert to sugar in your body and raise insulin levels as well. Too many grains are the same as too much sugar, with all of the same potential damages. Whole grains, while at least still containing fiber and nutrients, still lead to the same kinds of inflammatory, hormonal, weight gain type of issues as the sugar it turns into. Consciously limit these as well.

The only grains acceptable are sprouted, whole-grain, or stone-ground. These should still be used sparingly. Many people find they feel and do a whole lot better by nearly getting rid of grains altogether. Although it sounds tough, using almond, coconut, and flax flours, along with stevia and Xylitol® for sweeteners, you can make some amazing recipes that will easily replace breads and desserts in your home.

Remember that refined carbohydrates—such as flour, bread, and rice—turn into sugar almost immediately after putting them in your mouth as your saliva starts breaking them down. Don't be fooled. These foods are still sugar even if they don't taste sweet.

The good news is that if you cut sugar and grains, the cravings for them go away within a couple of weeks. Your sweet tooth can be easily managed with stevia and Xylitol®. Grains are replaced by almond, flax, and coconut flour. There are tons of great dessert and bread-like recipes to keep you happy on your health journey.

A lack of fiber is a real problem in the standard American diet. Refined products have the fiber removed. Pay careful attention to the high-fiber food lists and work more of them into your diet. Good fiber, not necessarily a packaged or pill version, is beneficial in your fight against all cancers—particularly those of the colon and other digestive organs.

Carbohydrates

Carbohydrates like fruits, vegetables, and grains are energy-producing foods. The higher a carbohydrate is on the glycemic index, however, the quicker it turns into sugar and upsets your hormone cycles. Eat a lot of high-glycemic and sugary foods and you're headed to insulin resistance, obesity, inflammation, and all the associated damages.

We know reducing or eliminating sugar intake can sound anywhere from tough to out of the question for you. But don't worry—there are a lot of options for dessert recipes and sweetening things up in the plan.

HEALTHY CARBOHYDRATES

GRAIN-FREE CARBOHYDRATE REPLACEMENTS: Flaxseed, almond flour, and coconut flour (and bread, muffins, crackers, and cookies made from them).

HIGH-FIBER/LOW-GLYCEMIC CARBOHYDRATES: High in fiber, these are always your best carbohydrate choices, any time of the day.

Vegetables: arugula, asparagus, bamboo shoots, bean sprouts, bell peppers (red, yellow, green), broad beans, broccoli, Brussels sprouts, cabbage, cassava, cauliflower, chives, celery, chayote fruit, chicory, coriander, collard greens, cucumber, eggplant, endive, fennel, garlic, ginger root, green beans, hearts of palm, jicama (raw), jalapeno peppers, kale, kohlrabi, lettuce, mushrooms, mustard greens, onions, parsley, radicchio, radishes, snap beans, snow peas, shallots, spinach, spaghetti squash, summer squash, Swiss chard, tomatoes, turnip greens, watercress, zucchini.

Fruits: Berries (Blackberries, Blueberries, Boysenberries, Elderberries, Gooseberries, Loganberries, Raspberries, Strawberries), Limes, Granny Smith Apples. Berries contain many Antioxidants, a lot of fiber and are the best fruits. Granny Smith Apples are low glycemic, thus have a minimal impact on blood sugar compared to other fruits.

MODERATE-FIBER/MODERATE-GLYCEMIC CARBOHYDRATES: Reduce consumption of these carbohydrates after lunch. Completely eliminate these carbohydrates after lunch if weight loss is a concern.

Vegetables and Grains: leeks, lima beans, okra, pumpkin, sweet potatoes or yams, turnips, legumes, artichokes, squash (acorn, butternut, winter), adzuki beans, black beans, chick peas (garbanzo), cowpeas, French beans, great northern beans, kidney beans, lentils, mung beans, navy beans, pinto beans, split peas, white beans, yellow beans, barley, brown rice, buckwheat (kasha), bulgar (tabouli), millet, steel-cut oats, rye, semolina, tapioca, whole grain breads, Ezekiel 4:9® bread, 100% whole-grain cooked cereals & crackers. Whether or not you're trying to lose weight, healthy grains are best used as an energy source when consumed early in the day. They shouldn't be eaten after lunch.

Fruits: cherries, pear, apricot, melons, orange, peach, plum, grapefruit, prunes, apples, kiwi, lemons, limes, nectarines, tangerines, passion fruit, persimmons, pomegranates.

HEALTHY CARBOHYDRATES

LOW-FIBER/HIGH-GLYCEMIC CARBOHYDRATES: Limit these. They contain a lot of sugar and, while natural, can still spike insulin. Best use is to eat these carbs as recovery from exercise. Avoid them completely if weight loss is a concern.

Vegetables, Tubers, and Grains: beets, carrots, corn, potatoes. Be cautious with carbohydrates and sugars from vegetables that are not grown above ground. They will alter insulin levels.

Fruits: bananas, pineapple, dates, grapes, watermelon, mangoes, papaya, honey, and fruit juices.

Vegetarianism

Vegetarianism is a popular approach to cancer prevention or treatment. A mostly raw diet that focuses on berries, vegetables, nuts, seeds, and beans, and not on grains is the proper approach if choosing this direction.

The Cancer Culprits

The following are some more examples of common foods in our diet that encourage the growth and proliferation of cancerous cells. (And no, it will not say that on the label.)

PROCESSED MEATS: This includes bacon, lunchmeat, hot dogs, packaged meats, sausage, and almost all frozen meats. After seven thousand clinical studies, The World Cancer Research Fund (WCRF) found that eating processed meats is directly linked to cancer. According to the WCRF website, "There is strong evidence that processed meats are causes of bowel cancer, and that there is no amount of processed meat that can be confidently shown not to increase risk." One of the main reasons processed meats are so dangerous is because they contain sodium nitrite, which helps give meat a red color, improves taste, and prevents spoilage. These Sodium Nitrites turn into nitrosamines, known carcinogens, in the body. A 2005 University of Hawaii study found that processed meats increase the risk of pancreatic cancer by 67 percent.[31] That is a risk not worth taking.

ACRYLAMIDES: These dangerous by-products come from heating foods at high temperatures (frying or grilling), and are found in high levels in potato chips, french fries, and cigarette smoke. According to the National Cancer Institute's website, "A series of case-control studies have investigated the relationship between dietary intake of acrylamide and the risk of developing cancers of the oral cavity, pharynx, esophagus, larynx, large bowel, kidney, breast, and ovary."

There is an easy solution to this barbecue dilemma. To avoid the formation of acrylamides in meats, marinate meat before cooking, which helps prevent the formation of acrylamides (use a combination of olive oil, lemon juice or apple cider vinegar, and anticancer spices like turmeric and garlic), and do not char the meat. It's better to cook longer at lower temperatures, away from the direct flame. If you're not familiar with some of these ingredients, consult your favorite barbecue master. They have all the secrets to a great grill!

ARTIFICIAL SWEETENERS: Aspartame (which is in Equal® and Nutrasweet®) has been linked to breast cancer. It contains phenylalanine, aspartic acid, and methanol (which break down into formaldehyde in the body). These are all potent neurotoxins. The American Cancer Society states that breast cancer rates have doubled since 1981. Not so coincidentally, that was the same year aspartame was approved for use in our food supply. Due to the Freedom of Information Act, records have now been made public that show that aspartame caused mammary tumors in rats tested by G.D. Searle (the maker of Nutrasweet® and Equal®) from 1971 to 1974, just before the FDA approval.[32] Dead rats tell no lies.

The newest sweetener, Splenda®, does not have any long-term studies to prove its safety, but it's a fact that it goes through an extensive chemical process (mostly involving chlorine, a commonly used chemical to sterilize swimming pools). So why wait for the studies? Stick with natural sweeteners, preferably stevia, as honey and agave nectar raise blood sugar.

PESTICIDES: Pesticides on produce, in animal feed, and residues in animal products and in our environment are known carcinogens, which can damage breast DNA and can disrupt or mimic normal hormonal activity.[33]

NON-ORGANIC ANIMAL PRODUCTS: Research shows that milk produced from cows treated with rBGH increases the risk for breast cancer and colon cancer. Nonorganic milk found on store shelves contains rBGH and other synthetics, which are known hormone disruptors. They can, for example, lead to circulating concentrations of insulin-like growth factor-1, thus increasing the risk of breast cancer.[34][35][36] Much of the farmed fish on the market (especially salmon and sea bass) contain high levels of PCBs (polychlorinated biphenyl) and dioxins, which are classified as persistent organic pollutants (POPs) and are known carcinogens. Although PCBs have been banned in the U.S. and in many other countries, many residues remain in our water supplies. Large fish at the top of the food chain pose an even higher health risk because of the bioaccumulation and concentration of PCBs.[37]

SOY: This so-called health food has been identified as a strong cancer-promoting food. According to Dr. Kayla Daniel, author of The Whole Soy Story, "The truth is that soy protein contains dangerous levels of plant estrogens. Although not identical to human estrogens, these compounds may mimic and/or disrupt the activity of estrogen within the body which may promote breast T-cell proliferation, a widely accepted marker of breast cancer risk."[38] Unfermented soy also contains phytates, which inhibit certain enzymes and interfere with thyroid function. Note: Not all soy products are unhealthy. Fermented soy like natto, miso, and tempeh boosts intestinal flora that help with digestion and immunity and contain an isoflavone known as genistein which has been demonstrated experimentally to have a broad range of chemopreventive properties.[39]

The Cancer Defenders

It is important to not only avoid the foods that compromise the body, but also to include the foods listed below to prevent cancer:

GREEN TEA: Green tea contains high levels of catechins, which can block the growth of cancers. According to Cancer Research UK, "They prevent DNA damage by mopping up free radicals, blocking the growth of tumor cells and stopping the activation of cancer-causing chemicals."[40]

BROCCOLI: One of the best cancer-fighting foods on the planet, it's loaded with various substances that fight or inhibit a wide range of cancers including breast, prostate, skin, colon and rectal cancers, and it does this in several different ways. It can promote the production of certain enzymes that deactivate free radicals and carcinogens and enable the body to detoxify dangerous hormone metabolites. One of these compounds, known as sulforaphane, which assists the body in metabolizing hormones, directly inhibits cancer cell proliferation and is found in up to one thousand times greater concentration in the sprouts of the broccoli versus the mature plant.

CABBAGE AND CAULIFLOWER: Like broccoli, these vegetables are members of the cruciferous family and are especially good at fighting breast cancer by converting cancer-promoting estrogens into a more protective type of hormone, i.e. conversion of estradiol into beneficial 2-hydroxyestrone versus harmful 16-hydroxyestrone.

CACAO: This raw form of chocolate is rich in flavanols, powerful antioxidants that are highly absorbable by the body. Cacao has a phenomenal oxygen radical absorbance capacity (ORAC). Caution: don't get too excited and load up on chocolate bars. This is not a free pass at the dessert counter, either. Most chocolate is loaded with other additives like milk products and sugar. Stick with raw cacao powder. Add it to smoothies and yogurt, or mix it with avocado and stevia for a mousse-like dessert.

DARK, LEAFY GREENS: Besides the incredible levels of vitamins, minerals, and fiber, dark, leafy greens like collards, escarole, kale, mustard greens, romaine lettuce, and Swiss chard are high in carotenoids and antioxidants, which inhibit the growth of certain types of breast cancer cells. Greens are also high in phytochemicals, which boost enzymes that detoxify carcinogens and help repair DNA damage to cells which can develop into cancer if left unchecked.

Dark leafy greens are a nutritional powerhouse that should be a regular part of everyone's diet.

ORGANIC ANIMAL PRODUCTS: (Wild caught fish, grass-fed beef, pasture raised poultry and eggs): Fish has high levels of omega-3 fatty acids and high levels of vitamin D, which is clearly a big player in breast cancer prevention. Grass-fed beef and organic butter have very high levels of conjugated linoleic acid (CLA) which is known to be a powerful cancer-fighting agent. Studies have shown that when human breast cancer cells were incubated in high CLA milk fat, the growth of the cancer cells decreased by 90 percent.[41] A French study also showed that women with the highest CLA levels had a 74% lower risk of developing breast cancer.[42]

CURCUMIN: This power-packed spice found in curry powder and turmeric contains compounds that protect against breast cancer and tumor growth. Simply add it to soups, spreads, smoothies, salads, etc.

FLAXSEED: This is one of the most powerful anticancer foods known, and one of the only seeds that has been found to inhibit and/or regress cancer in human clinical studies. In 2005, the journal Clinical Cancer Research published a placebo-controlled study involving patients who received daily a 25-gram flaxseed-containing muffin over the course of thirty-two days. After observing a reduction in tumor markers and an increase in programmed cell death (apoptosis) in the flaxseed-treated patients, the authors concluded: "Dietary flaxseed has the potential to reduce tumor growth in patients with breast cancer."[43] Treatment of prostate cancer, another hormone-sensitive cancer, has also benefited from this remarkable seed. In a 2008 study published in the journal Cancer Epidemiology, Biomarkers & Prevention, men who received flaxseed for twenty-one days before prostate surgery had significantly reduced cancer proliferation rates in their prostates.[44]

CARROTS: High in beta carotene, carrots fight many forms of cancer including lung, stomach, intestinal, bladder, prostate, breast, throat and mouth. It's better to eat them raw rather than cooked and in moderation due to high sugar content.

MUSHROOMS: Many varieties, such as versicolor, coriolus, murill, agaricus blazei, reishi, maitake, and shiitake, contain powerful immune-boosting polysaccharides, such as beta-glucan, which can enhance the natural killer cell count and activity in such a way that directly inhibits cancer cell proliferation. This category has been extensively researched, and there are human clinical studies published in peer-reviewed medical journals demonstrating improved survival and outcomes using mushroom extracts in cancer treatment.

SEAWEED: This contains beta carotene, as well as the cancer-fighting carotenoid fucoxanthin, and is high in other key nutrients that are of great value to immune health.

ORGANIC AND FERMENTED SOY: Despite mainstream misconceptions, soy is not bad for your health if it's organic, and especially when fermented. In Asia, the incidences of many cancers that afflict the West are reduced, if not altogether nonexistent.

TOMATOES: It's one of the anticancer super foods that contains lycopene, and is high in antioxidants that attack the cancer-triggering free radicals in the body. Lycopene is known to kill mouth cancer cells and is linked to reduced risk of breast, prostate, pancreas and colorectal cancers. It's actually more effective cooked than raw.

AVOCADOS: They're high in antioxidants. It's now believed that they may be useful in treating viral hepatitis, which causes liver cancer, as well as other types of liver damage.

CITRUS FRUITS: Including grapefruit, oranges, and lemons, help to remove carcinogens from the body, preventing various cancers. They may also stimulate cancer-killing immune cells. They're high in vitamin C and beta carotene.

BERRIES: Strawberries, raspberries and blueberries have been shown to help prevent cancers of the skin, bladder, lung and breast, largely because of their ellagic acid content. All are high in antioxidants, but the anthocyanosides in blueberries are the most powerful known in science.

NUTS: They're high in antioxidants. Brazil nuts in particular help against prostate cancer because of their highly bio-available and therapeutic form of selenium.

Additional Supplements

Unfortunately, much of what we need to be healthy, and even to prevent breast cancer, simply can't be obtained through our current diets. While you should never take more than you need, there are some fundamental essentials that just about everyone needs on a daily basis to stay healthy.

ESSENTIAL FATTY ACIDS: omega-3s and healthy omega-6s are crucial to long-term health and to ward off the onset of cancer. (More on omegas in Chapter 13).

QUALITY MULTIVITAMINS: Don't go cheap here, and it's good to go with gender-specific formulas. An inexpensive, common drug or grocery store brand will likely detract from and not add to your wellness. You want to find a third-party tested, all-natural product from a reputable company.

VITAMIN D: Vitamin D is produced in the body when the sun interacts with your skin. Unfortunately, Americans are spending much less time in the sun and when they do, they're loading up on sunscreen. As a result, most people are alarmingly deficient in vitamin D. Recent studies show that ideal serum vitamin D levels should be at or above 80ng/ml to take advantage of the cancer preventive and overall health benefits of vitamin D. Another recent study showed that a serum vitamin D level of 52ng/mL reduces breast cancer risk by 83 percent.[45] Similar studies have shown that higher levels of vitamin D drastically reduce the likelihood of cancers to spread. In order to get serum levels up to the ideal range, most people need supplementation. Maintenance doses are 5,000 IU, but some people may need to take more to get their levels up to the ideal levels.[46]

The Essentials from Cancer-Killing Essential No. 3

1. Increase your intake of healthy fats and eliminate the bad fats.

2. Moderate your intake of protein. Animal products are the most important foods to buy organic and naturally raised. On average, men should consume 20 grams of protein per meal, and women should consume 15 grams of protein per meal. Consume 5 to 10 additional grams of protein after exercise.

3. Reduce or eliminate grains and sugars, and limit fruits to the morning, trying to stick mainly with berries, Granny Smith Apples or grapefruit.

4. Avoid the "Culprits."

5. Consume some of the "Defenders" at each meal.

6. At a minimum, take the basic supplements – Vitamin D3, Omegas, and a quality multivitamin.

CHAPTER 10
CANCER-KILLING ESSENTIAL NO. 4: MAXIMIZED OXYGEN & LEAN MUSCLE

How much lean muscle you have compared to body fat matters for more than dress sizes and Speedos. Better lean muscle to body fat ratios play a big role in overall health.

Oxygen is a more important elemental nutrient for survival than any nutrient you can swallow. Oxygen has been shown to stymie the growth of cancers. Healthy cells love oxygen, and cancer cells hate it. It makes sense, doesn't it? (Remember: cancer's preferred source of fuel is sugar.)

Essential No. 4: Maximized Oxygen and Lean Muscle (through exercise) is a major step in attending to cancer causes.

The far-too-sedentary American lifestyle represents one of the deadliest carcinogens out there. Our couch-potatoism leads to obesity, and as we mentioned in Essential No. 3, extra fat leaves your body more susceptible to cancer. In addition, lack of exercise, no matter what your weight, still puts you at a higher risk for cancer.

Building muscle and losing fat diminishes your chances of developing cancer of any type. For example, a study of thirteen thousand men and women followed for fifteen years by aerobics guru, Dr. Kenneth Cooper, showed that poor diet and lack of exercise caused as much as 60% of all colorectal cancers in men and 40% in women. Out-of-shape people were shown to be 300% more likely to develop cancer.

CANCERS DIRECTLY LINKED TO LACK OF EXERCISE:

• Breast (among women who have gone through menopause)

• Colon and Rectum

• Endometrium (lining of the uterus)

• Esophagus

• Kidney

• Pancreas

BEING OVERWEIGHT MAY ALSO RAISE THE RISK OF OTHER CANCERS:[47]

• Gallbladder

• Liver

• Non-Hodgkin Lymphoma

• Multiple Myeloma

• Cervix

• Ovary

• Aggressive forms of prostate cancer

THE POWERFUL EFFECT OF A PROPERLY APPLIED EXERCISE PROGRAM ON PHYSIOLOGY IS THE KEY REASON FOR ITS CANCER-STOPPING EFFECTS. EXERCISE IMPROVES:

• Cardiovascular capacity

• Lung capacity

• Circulation

• Immune function, such as an increase in white blood cells, interleukin or neutrophils

• Speed and function of bowel motility

• Antioxidant defenses

• Ideal hormone levels

The right kind of physical training lowers bad hormone levels, increases good ones, boosts immune functions, helps manage weight, and lowers body fat, all of which are known causes of breast cancer. The simple conclusion is that lack of exercise causes malfunction and interferes with the body's ability to kill the enemy.

Exercise and Hormones

Growth hormone (GH) and testosterone help build muscle and burn fat. Both GH and testosterone decline naturally with age, but that can be overcome by ramping them back up with exercise.

Exercise done at the right duration and intensity can increase these good hormone levels for hours or even days. Exercise also helps to optimize Estrogen and Thyroid hormone. These two hormones have not only been connected to cancer, but also impact metabolism, fat-to-muscle ratios, mood, and sex drive. By regulating these hormones, you look better, prevent disease, and like sex more. So everyone wins.

With quality fitness, blood levels of the fat hormone Insulin decrease and the cells regain their Insulin sensitivity. Keeping Insulin in check is critical to cancer killing on so many levels, as mentioned in the Essential No. 3 section.

The Right Kind of Exercise Program

Pay attention to the three Ts: Time, Tempo, and Type. How long you exercise, the tempo or intensity, and the type of exercises you're performing are very important. These three Ts can greatly influence the impact you can have on your hormone production.

The good news is that shorter, more intense intervals make the most difference in helping your body's physiology improve. So while you have to push it and get your heart rate up, it's only for brief periods of time. This kind of daily workout seen in surge training and interval training can be done in as little as twelve minutes. We use the MaxT3 program developed by Maximized Living to easily apply this.

Studies also show that exercising less than three days per week is ineffective. Some type of rigorous movement should be attempted almost daily. But more is not always better when it comes to cancer prevention. Some research says there is a diminishing rate of return when you exceed moderate daily levels. This is another great reason to keep your exercise sessions short and sweet—but intense, so you get the desired physiological results.

Deep breathing throughout the day is another good method of maximizing oxygen. Unfortunately, most Americans take extremely shallow breaths during most of the day. To achieve proper deep breathing, learn by watching a baby. As babies breathe in through their noses, their abdomens will extend considerably. This utilizes both the upper and lower lungs. As we get older, life pulls us away from this natural deep breathing. By consciously breathing deeply on a regular basis, you'll raise the levels of oxygen within the blood. Again, this creates a happy home for good cells and an unsuitable home for cancers. On a cellular level, it is possible that cancer may be attacked at its root. Note: Deep breathing is also a great technique for stress reduction.

Proof of the Power of Movement

BREAST CANCER: A study of 2,296 women with stages I, II, and III breast cancer was performed by researchers at the Brigham and Women's Hospital and Harvard Medical School, both in Boston. They found that the risk of death from breast cancer fell 19% for those who walked or did similar exercises for one to three hours per week and by 54% for those working out three to five hours per week.[48]

OVARIAN CANCER: A study of more than 2,100 women found that those who exercised more than six hours per week were 27% less likely to develop ovarian cancer than women who exercised less than one hour each week, according to an October 2000 article in the *Journal Obstetrics and Gynecology*.[49]

ENDOMETRIAL CANCER: Four hours of housework or a brisk sixty-minute walk alone can reduce endometrial cancer risk by 30%, according to researchers from the Vanderbilt University Medical Center in Nashville, Tennessee, and the Shanghai

Cancer Institute in China. (Findings presented at the 95th Annual Meeting of the American Association for Cancer Research in Orlando, Florida, on March 29, 2004).

OVERALL INCIDENCE IN MEN: A 2004 Danish research project that followed five thousand men over a twenty-three-year period established the role fitness plays in cancer prevention. The Copenhagen Male Study was able to attribute moderate physical activity to boosting the function of the immune system, according to reports. Higher immune function promotes cancer prevention.[50]

PROSTATE CANCER: The hormonal and immune impacting voltage created by exercise puts all the indicators in place to support men's efforts to thwart prostate cancer. One recent study suggested that regular, vigorous activity could slow the progression of prostate cancer in men sixty-five or older.[51]

COLON CANCER: Fitness has been shown to reduce the risk of colon cancer—but why? One likely reason is that exercise speeds up the rate at which waste moves through the body, offering less carcinogenic exposure. A Harvard University study followed seventeen thousand alumni over twenty-five years and showed that the group of men that were highly active, using up at least 2,500 calories per week exercising about forty-five minutes per day, experienced half the incidences of colon cancer when compared with the sedentary group.

Note: Multiple studies around the world have regularly shown that adults, by increasing physical activity in virtually any way, can reduce their risk of contracting colon cancer by 30 to 40 percent. The greatest risk reduction is seen among those who are the most active.[52 53 54 55]

LUNG CANCER: Physical activity, even just the fun stuff like yoga or planting a garden, is inversely related to mortality from respiratory diseases, including lung cancer. Many studies point to the fact that the benefits work for everyone whether or not they smoked, were a former smoker, or never touched the stuff. More good news is that exercise improves survival rates for those diagnosed with lung cancer![56 57 58 59]

RECOVERING FROM CANCER: : If you currently have a cancer diagnosis or have had it in the past, you should aim to conquer it the same way you prevent it. Exercise is still the wonder treatment. All of the positive physiological impacts of rigorous activity are critical to prevent, deal with, and/or recover from cancer.[60 61] For more information see the book, Cancer Prevention and Management Through Exercise and Weight Control, edited by Anne McTiernan.

CHAPTER 11

CANCER KILLING ESSENTIAL NO. 5: MINIMIZED TOXINS

There are many practical ways to make fitness and nutrition fit into your life, but what do you do when you realize that cancer is caused by your environment? How do you escape all the toxins around you every day in the air, in the water, on public buses and airplanes, in your car, the pesticides your neighbors use on their lawn, in home cleaning solutions, and in your shampoo, sunscreen, and toothpaste? Do you have to move to a far away, cleaner country and live off the land?

It's not so easy. The solution isn't moving: You literally can't get away from it. There's nowhere to go to escape toxins. Even if you travel to the most desolate place in Antarctica or deep into the jungles of Peru, you'll still find cancer-causing chemicals. You'll find them in the water, the soil, and the air. You'll find toxins in the breast milk, bloodstreams, and urine samples of the inhabitants there, many of which we know will cause cells to mutate and can develop into cancer.

Why don't we hear more about this? Food producers, product manufacturers, government officials, pharmaceutical companies, medical physicians and others will admit that while the chemicals present in products could be harmful in high doses, they're perfectly safe in the small amounts that a product contains. And if we were exposed only once in our lives, that might be a meaningful statement. The problem is we are exposed over and over again to these chemicals and eventually they build up in our systems.

While you aren't likely to get cancer from one injection at your pediatrician's office, one diet cola, one cigarette, one order of fast food, the new car smell, or one application of chemically-based skin lotion, these toxic materials cannot be effectively metabolized by your body. Therefore, these poisons accumulate or build up in your system and create what is called a "toxic burden." This gradual buildup of toxins in your blood, cells, tissues or organs can go undetectable for years until symptoms start to become obvious. Over time, the burden becomes too great for the body to carry. So while they don't cause disease or death today, they most certainly can tomorrow.

As toxins accumulate, they interfere with normal cell life and cause the cells in the body to react to the rising levels of unwelcome agents. As this occurs, symptoms linked to the toxicity and new, mysterious illnesses such as Chronic Fatigue Syndrome and Fibromyalgia begin to pop up while incidences of disorders like depression, Attention Deficit Disorder (ADD) and Attention Deficit Hyperactivity Disorder (ADHD) rise. Other examples of toxin-linked conditions include asthma, which is 10 times more prevalent in children now than at the beginning of the decade: Sleeplessness, weight loss resistance, early onset of puberty, Thyroid failure, Parkinson's, Alzheimer's, and of course, cancer.

These toxins really attack both Supersystems – the Central Nervous System and the Immune System. They infiltrate the body on many levels, being stored not only outside the cells in the blood and tissues, but also inside the cells. Where they store and accumulate over time, they cause damage.

WHAT TOXINS ARE OUT THERE AND WHERE THEY ARE FOUND

Plastics

Fruits and vegetables are healthy, right? Not necessarily—not if they're wrapped in plastic, as virtually everything is nowadays. Each day we eat so many foods that come in contact with plastics and phthalate (a substance added to plastic to make it more flexible) that the government has actually established an average daily amount that we can safely ingest.

Drinking out of plastic water bottles or microwaving food in plastic containers exposes you to very high levels of phthalates and other chemicals.

Plastics damage hormone receptors, hurt sex drive, cause fatigue, harm brain chemistry, accumulate in organs, and lead to illness. They've been specifically linked to cancers of the prostate, breast, lung, and thyroid.

Many plastics also contain bisphenol A (BPA), which has become extremely controversial and is illegal in some countries. Scientists are concerned that BPA, a xenoestrogen, is linked to certain types of cancer, lowered levels of testosterone, and other serious health effects like obesity, attention deficits, lowered sperm counts, and can cause early puberty onset. Problems can occur even at low doses.

Another chemical our foods come in contact with is polystyrene. The Styrofoam trays that many foods sit in contain the toxin polystyrene, which is made from the chemical styrene. Phthalate and styrene chemicals leach more aggressively into foods and liquids when heated. Think about that as you drink your hot coffee from a Styrofoam cup tomorrow morning.

Environment

Every chemical named in this chapter makes its way into the environment in one way or another. The ground in which our foods are grown and the grass in which we play contain many layers of chemicals and pesticides used to kill things. Birds suffer from these poisons as do small animals. Why would we think they would not affect us as well? We spread these chemicals on our lawns and then days later we let our children play on the same grass. Even if time has passed, these chemicals linger.

Environmental endocrine disruptors (EEDs) are toxins that imitate hormones. By blocking or altering hormone functions, they can lead to an increase in hormone-related cancers, such as those of the breast, testicles and prostate, which are all not coincidentally on the rise. Endocrine disruptors can be found everywhere in chemicals like phthalates, dioxins, pesticides, detergents, polystyrene and trichloroethylene and in most households and garage cleaning and maintenance supplies. Worse still, it can be found in tap water.

Dioxins are an example of these EEDs. They're indigestible and therefore accumulate in the body. Dioxins are created through the manufacturing of plastics, pesticides, and other chemicals that end up in our foods and beverages. These chemicals are a potent cause of cancer. Through breast milk, infants can consume up to eighteen times more carcinogenic dioxin in one year than the maximum "safe" lifetime dose as recommended by the U.S. Centers for Disease Control and Prevention in Atlanta, Georgia, the federal agency charged with protecting public health.

Of course, the companies that make these products and the governmental agencies that approve them claim that they're present in such minuscule amounts that they aren't harmful. The problem, once again, is that these so-called miniscule amounts accumulate until they become toxic time bombs.

Water

You have to watch what you drink, bathe in, and what you use to clean and prepare foods. Tap water is full of chlorine, heavy metals, contaminants, and other toxins. Chlorine is a big one. If it's strong enough to kill bacteria and other dangerous stuff in our water, do you really think it's a good idea to drink it? And it doesn't end at chlorine and heavy metals.

Many studies have found prescription drugs, including beta blockers, estrogen, antidepressants, and pain killers in tap water. Not surprisingly, a 2006 article in the International Journal of Cancer concluded that drinking tap water left men, in particular, as much as 50% more vulnerable to bladder cancer. With this knowledge in hand, it's up to you to decide whether or not to drink it and in what quantity.[62]

Benzene

One of the chemicals we highly suspect was involved with Dr. Majors' condition was benzene, which is frequently linked with leukemia. It's found in auto exhaust, gasoline, plastics, rubbers, dyes, detergents, carpets, pesticides, and some drugs. Dr. Majors had lived in several new homes and had built multiple clinics. Building materials and home furnishings are loaded with hazardous materials that, particularly when new, expel harmful gases into the environment and end up stuck in people's bodies.

Even though he was taking great care of himself in the years before his diagnosis, heavy exposure and damage from benzene and a host of other chemicals would trump healthy lifestyle, if not directly addressed.

The following is an important list of chemicals and where they're found. Take this problem seriously and reduce your exposure, and work to eliminate as many as you can from your system. The point is to think about what you choose to consume and use. Read the labels and opt for products that offer the lowest exposure to these harmful elements.

Heavy Metal Poisons

Cadmium, aluminum, mercury, antimony, lead, and arsenic are all heavy metals we get from manufactured products, industry run-off, dentistry (amalgam fillings), medications, vaccinations, pesticides, manufacturing, aviation, the auto industry, and auto and industrial exhaust. They're also present in personal hygiene products, appliances, and aluminum-lined boxes and cans. Food additives also contain heavy metals.

Heavy metals are known as neurotoxins, meaning they can poison the central nervous system. They're linked to many types of chronic neurological disorders.

Your Own Mouth

One of the first places to look for Neurotoxins from heavy metals and bacteria is in your mouth. For Dr. Majors, this was another significant factor in his cancer. Look at three areas:

1. AMALGAM FILLINGS: Slowly leak Mercury and other metals that are very toxic.

2. ROOT CANALS: Allow patients to keep a "dead tooth" in their mouth, which can devastate the human Immune System. When the dentist removes the bulk of the nerve from the root canal, he cannot treat the millions of Tubules with dead nerve tissue that remain. There are about three miles of these Tubules with dead debris in the average tooth. That's three miles of possible infection. It is better to lose a dead tooth.

3. CAVITATIONS: While a Cavity is a hole in the tooth, a cavitation is a hole in the bone that is not in plain sight. These lesions are often located in old extraction sites (especially of molars and wisdom teeth), and under or near the roots of root canal teeth or dead teeth. They can spread from these locations throughout the jawbone and may penetrate the sinuses or totally encompass the jaw nerve. Research shows that all cavitation tissue samples tested contain toxins, which significantly inhibit one or more of five basic body enzymes necessary in the energy production cycle. There are indications that when these toxins combine with chemicals or heavy metals, such as fluoride or mercury, more potent toxins may be formed.

Food Additives

Stay away from foods containing food additives, dyes, colorings, flavorings, stabilizers, fake fats, artificial sugars, and preservatives. The average person ingests 140 to 150 pounds of additives every year.[63]

Medications

The nearly four billion prescription drugs, over-the-counter medicines, and vaccines are themselves chemical toxins. Additionally, phthalates, heavy metals, and commercial preservatives are used to both coat the drugs and preserve the materials. Vaccines, for example, contain a multitude of chemicals, preservatives, and heavy metals such as formaldehyde, aluminum, phosphates, sodium chloride, sodium hydroxide, hydrochloride, sorbitol, and hydrolyzed gelatin that are unsafe at any dose, but are injected into our bloodstreams by the dozens as part of normal childhood "wellness" protocols.

Personal Care Products

These toxins are literally hiding in plain sight on the shelves and in the drawers in your bathroom. They're in your shower and by your sink. You wash with them and use them to make yourself more beautiful, and to make yourself smell better. The list includes sunscreens, makeup, skin creams and lotions, soaps, shampoos, bubble baths, laundry and dishwashing detergents, and toothpastes. And they all contain harmful chemicals that you gladly smear on your skin, scrub on your teeth, or spray on your hair.

DIETHANOLAMINE: Also known as DEA, is among the most prolific of the carcinogens found in personal care products. It serves as a wetting agent in a huge number of products, giving shampoos their rich lather and lotions their creamy consistency. It has been labeled as carcinogenic by the National Toxicology Program and the International Agency for Research on Cancer. Particularly when mixed with a nitroso compound, it has been proven to be carcinogenic in a variety of lab animals and has been banned in parts of Europe. In 1995 the National Institute of Environmental Health Sciences described DEA as having low acute toxicity, but significant cumulative toxicity.

SODIUM LAURYL SULFATE: Is a common degreaser used in practically every soap, shampoo, and toothpaste on the market today. The compound has been used in studies to induce mutation in bacteria and irritate skin. It has also shown to enter the heart, liver, lungs and brain from skin contact, and has been proven to maintain residual levels once inside these organs.

FLUORIDE: Added to the nation's drinking water and toothpaste, purportedly to protect children's teeth from tooth decay, is a halogen that can cause cell membrane damage and hormone issues. This has been linked to behavioral disorders, birth defects, flu, and arthritis. Fluoride can also cause damage to the heart, brain, and kidneys. It can interfere with metabolism of testosterone. Scientists have also challenged whether research even backs its role in preventing tooth decay.

PROPYLENE GLYCOL: This one makes the rounds of households concealed in antifreeze solutions and hydraulic fluids as a powerful solvent. Astonishingly, it's also found in childhood vaccinations, cosmetics, toothpastes, shampoos, deodorants, lotions, and even processed foods, including pet foods. It has been found to cause problems like kidney damage, liver abnormalities, skin cell growth inhibition, damaged cell membranes, rashes, respiratory damage, immune system deficiency, and central nervous system depression.

This is only a partial list of the literally thousands of chemicals being slipped into food and products, given the opportunity to enter our bodies and then allowed to accumulate there for years to come.

Home/Work

There are too many chemicals in carpets and carpet cleaners to list. Add to that: **TOLUENE** in paints; **PHTHALATES** in wallpaper, dishes, tablecloths, and shower curtains; **FORMALDEHYDE** in pressed wood kitchen cabinets, wood preservatives, furniture, and mattress fabrics; and **XYLENE** in towels and blankets.

Children's playthings, including the very baby bottles, rattles, and teething toys they eagerly shove into their mouths, are often made from unhealthy plastics and, in rarer cases, neurotoxic metals.

Teflon cookware contains **PERFLUOROOCTANOIC ACID**, a known carcinogen commonly found in people's bloodstreams.

PHENOL is another extremely common chemical present in plywood, disinfectants, medical products, food, and auto emissions, and has been linked to Breast Cancer.

Yard

Pesticides, insecticides, herbicides, molluscosides, fungicides, and fertilizers are abundant at home and in the fields and parks where children and pets play.

Car

Car exhaust contains hydrocarbons, formaldehyde, and benzene. That's why you can't shut the garage and stay in the car while it's running, but you're living in it during rush hour.

These are just some of the chemicals we're exposed to every day. We left out dry cleaning, silicone breast implants, and titanium hip replacements. To keep things simple, you'd be safe to assume that almost every product has some chemicals with the potential to give you cancer and that prospect should be truly frightening.

ADDRESS THE CAUSE, REMOVE THE INTERFERENCE: CANCER KILLERS NEED TO PROTECT AND DETOXIFY

Minimize Exposure

After reading this long list of everyday toxic substances, you can see that trying to avoid man-made chemicals entirely would be an impossible task. But through awareness, you can at least limit exposure.

You also have important detox pathways like your lungs, liver, colon, and kidneys that are capable of managing some amount of foreign chemicals daily. By minimizing exposure and applying the Five Essentials, you do a lot to help these pathways manage toxic levels.

One of the major concerns with all of the toxins listed above is that children are exposed to them like never before, and as we've said, they accumulate rapidly. Studies on umbilical cord blood show a significant toxic load from the mothers. Never before have we been exposed to so many toxins from birth.

Detoxifying Toxins

Your body can't metabolize the bulk of these poisons. They bio-accumulate, and eventually the toxic burden will become far too great for your detox pathways. Because these chemicals are incredibly prevalent in your daily life, you need to intentionally make sure you're detoxifying them.

Detoxifying involves more than a colon cleanse. Toxins bind to the inside of cells and get stored outside the cells in fats and tissues. On top of that, they're specifically eliminated by certain nutrients and detox pathways that will diminish and begin shutting down upon constant chemical bombardment.

Inside the Cell

For intracellular detoxification, you need to turn to your body's own natural antioxidant, glutathione, which exists to get toxins out from inside the cell.[64] It's utilized by virtually every cell in your body to maintain cellular health and prevent the proliferation of harmful free radicals. Naturally, to aid detoxification, glutathione levels are highest in the liver and kidneys, which are the body's primary detoxification organs.

A bombardment of toxins causes your body's stores of glutathione to run down. If this happens, you're less capable of dealing with environmental toxins and less able to remove them from your body. This is why one person can walk into an office that smells of perfume, mold, or fresh paint and be un-phased, while another person is hammered by the toxins in the air and goes into a full migraine headache for three days.

You can get glutathione by eating foods that contain it, supplements built from these foods, intravenously, as a compound breathed through a nebulizer, or by taking glycine, glutamic acid, and cysteine—which are the building blocks of glutathione—so your body can manufacture it on its own.

Vegetables that contain higher levels of glutathione include spinach, broccoli, and carrots. It's vital to consume them raw on a regular basis. Cooking vegetables depletes their usable glutathione contents by nearly 100 percent. There is some glutathione available in properly raised meat, dairy, and eggs. But again, these sources are only significant when the foods are in their raw forms.[65]

Green foods are critical. Green, leafy vegetables in the form of salads, juices, and supplements contain powerful enzymes, key proteins, and chlorophyll, which is the ultimate purification molecule for the body. Additional antioxidant enzymes like glutathione that are important to reduce oxidative stress within the cells are superoxide dismutase (SOD) and catalase. SOD has also been used to treat long-term damage from exposure to smoke and radiation, prevent side effects from cancer medications, and for treating inflammatory diseases.

These free-radical-scavenging enzymes guard your cells. Getting them in your diet is difficult and would likely require supplementation. Additionally, vitamins (B2, B6, and selenium) are necessary for glutathione synthesis in the body, so eating foods rich in these nutrients, or getting them through supplements, is helpful.

Other sulfur-rich compounds like glutathione that bind toxins for inter-cell removal are vitamin U, cultured dairy proteins, and whey proteins (lactalbumin).

Outside the Cell

To remove toxins from the extracellular tissues, pure water and high-fiber foods help to flush the body of toxicity. High-fiber foods do this by literally grabbing toxins and removing them. The best are soft fiber foods like fruits, some vegetables, and a great, detoxifying food rich in fiber, healthy fats and vitamins called avocado.

Because of gut damage and its impact on digestion, elimination, and detox pathway function you need to get probiotics from either cultured dairy products or a high quality probiotic supplement.

Another necessity for proper extracellular toxin elimination is activated charcoal. If you call poison control, they would tell you that charcoal is one of the best elements out there for binding up the poisons from the system and allowing for safe elimination. Charcoal is available in supplement form. As with all supplements, the type, quantity, and how and when it's applied are very important.

The best detoxifying phytochemicals are broccoli and others in the brassica/ cruciferous family of vegetables, such as Brussels sprouts, cauliflower, kale, collard greens, watercress, turnips, horseradish, and cilantro. All aid in detoxification. Caution: the body's ability to use nutrients and supplements is directly proportional to their quality. Invest here in the fresh and organic, so you're not investing in medicine later.

ANOTHER WAY TO DETOX: FAR INFRARED SAUNA

Your body also has the ability to get rid of toxins in your sweat. Infrared sauna has been found to be a good way to speed up the poison elimination process.

In reaction to becoming heated in an infrared sauna, your body's core temperature increases. Heating up the body triggers your sweat mechanism. From there, your body can dump chemicals through its largest organ—your skin.

The theory behind far infrared heat is that it directly penetrates the body's tissues at a depth greater than a regular sauna. While a conventional sauna or steam room relies only on indirect heat from the surrounding air, far infrared heat is also creating heat within the body. This internal body heat will cause toxins deeper within the cells and tissues to be driven out.

CHAPTER 12
THE "DON'T GET IT " PLAN

It's not just your body and your life you need to be concerned about. Many others love you and are counting on you. Accept responsibility and take charge of your lifestyle and how your body is functioning and healing.

It's not that hard. We've put together a plan that will address the causes and remove the interference of disease. If you have cancer, then this "Don't Get It" plan has even more urgency as a "Get Rid of It" plan. You'll go beyond this plan when you get to the next chapters where we're giving you even more weapons in your arsenal to overcome this symptom called cancer.

Millions of people, in some way, shape, or form are following the Don't Get It Plans of this world and taking a stand. They are the Cancer Killers.

Putting the Five Essentials into Practice

Here is a simple checklist of Dos and Don'ts from the Five Essentials.

ESSENTIAL NO. 1:

- Forgive. Forgive yourself and others. Forgiveness is a way of letting go of anger and hurt, and in the end improves your health and the function of your immune system. You're not forgiving to let the other person off the hook; you're forgiving so you can live healthier, free of the stress and duress anger causes. The Stanford University Center for Research in Disease Prevention reported that holding onto bitterness for an extended period of time "wears out your immune system and hurts your heart."[66]

- If there is a problem with someone or something, confront it like an adult. Don't let it fester.

- Take care of yourself. Maybe you have children or older relatives to care for, but you need to take weekly time for yourself.

- Take responsibility for your life. Never assume problems are outside of your control.

- Become a Possibility Thinker. When you believe something is possible, you put yourself in a position to win.

ESSENTIAL NO. 2:

- Find a corrective care chiropractor to ensure proper communication between your brain and body.

- Do your daily spinal corrective exercises.

ESSENTIAL NO. 3:

- Increase your intake of healthy fats.

- Moderate your intake of protein. Animal products are the most important foods to keep organic. An average man should consume 20 grams of protein per meal, and a woman should consume 15 grams of protein per meal. Consume five to ten additional grams of protein after exercise.

- Reduce or eliminate grains and sugars, and limit fruits, trying to stick mainly with berries or Granny Smith apples. Use stevia and Xylitol® to sweeten.

- Avoid the "Culprits."

- Utilize the "Defenders" at each meal.

- At a minimum, take the basic supplements, including Vitamin D, Omegas, and a quality multivitamin.

ESSENTIAL NO. 4:

- Exercise to increase the flow of oxygen.

- Do short-duration, high-intensity workouts a minimum of three days each week and some type of rigorous movement six days per week.

- Do deep breathing throughout the day to raise the oxygen levels present in the blood.

ESSENTIAL NO. 5:

- Eat foods and take a detox supplement(s) daily that can pull toxins out from both inside and outside the cells. This is so you can guard against the daily bombardment of toxins.

- Avoid all body care products that contain ingredients that you can't pronounce or couldn't eat (in small quantities).

- Buy organic whenever possible, especially when it comes to meat and dairy.

- Get blood tests that check for the presence of dangerous chemicals and heavy metals like mercury.

The key to never getting cancer is to be a Cancer Killer every day! Most blood testing as well as medical screening (mammograms, CT scans, etc.) are early detection systems for disease. When they find something, it means you already have cancer. That's not prevention; that's containment!

Because all of us are human, we make mistakes and are constantly surrounded by carcinogenic toxins. So it's important to do more than just test to see if cancer is there. There are important markers that tell you not only whether you have a full-blown diagnosis already, but whether your body is on its way to this disease. If you detect cancer early, even before it's a full blown medical crisis, you can become more aggressive and specific in your protocols.

With the exception of blood cancers, blood tests will never absolutely tell you whether or not you have cancer, but blood tests can give you and your doctor clues about what's going on inside your body.

Practitioners of conventional medicine will rarely run some of these tests without full-blown symptoms! Why? Because if a patient is in a very early stage of cancer, they have nothing they can do to help, unless you want dangerous chemotherapy and radiation. So here is a list of blood tests and virus tests that you should ask for.

Begin with a basic CBC blood and then add these additional blood tests and virus tests listed below. If any of your blood work is abnormal, you need to consult with someone who is qualified to evaluate the results.

BLOOD TESTS TO ADD:

- LDH (lactate dehydrogenase)

- IGF-binding Protein - III

- ESR (erythrocyte sedimentation rate)

- Iron serum magnesium (RBC)

- Ferritin serum calcium

- Transferrin saturation (%)

- TIBC (total iron binding capacity)

- Vitamin D (1,25 DI-OH & 25 OH-VIT D)

- Hemoglobin A1C

- CRP/homocysteine

ADDITIONAL TEST FOR UNDERLYING VIRUSES AND INFECTIOUS AGENTS:

- H-Pylori

- EBV

- Hepatitis B and C

- CMV

- HPV

- HSV

- HIV

Underlying Viruses

Professor Robert Souhami, Director Of Clinical Research for Cancer Research UK, said that between 15% and 20% of all cancers are caused by viruses.[67] We believe it's much higher than that!

So how are viruses a cause of cancer? A virus is nothing more than DNA or RNA wrapped in a protein coating. They can't survive on their own; they have to invade a nearby cell in order to survive and grow. There are two ways an underlying virus can cause cancer:

1. The virus invades a nearby cell and alters the cell's genetic coding, causing a mutation. This mutation can result in cancer.

2. The virus preoccupies the immune system so it can't do a proper job killing off cancer. In other words, the immune system is temporarily overwhelmed.

Here are some of the viruses you need to address: EBV, HPV, Herpes, HIV, CMV, and Hepatitis B and C. There are many other viruses that could contribute to causing cancer as well, but these pose the biggest challenge to the body.

If your blood test reveals you have a virus, you need to address it immediately, because it will overwhelm the immune system pretty quickly. Most viruses, like cancer, are anaerobic, which means they hate oxygen and can't exist in an elevated oxygen environment. So by increasing cellular oxygen levels, you prevent these viruses from replicating, proliferating, and ultimately, from existing.

Ozone blood cleaning and UVB blood cleaning are used by a lot of natural doctors to help with getting rid of the underlying virus. And don't forget Essential No. 4 for creating a more oxygen sufficient and efficient body.

CHAPTER 13
TOP SUPER SUPPLEMENTS AND TOP NONTOXIC TREATMENTS

The U.S. Food and Drug Administration is charged with evaluating new drugs to determine whether clinical trials prove that medications do what their manufacturers claim, and what side-effect risks they pose. The agency's job is to protect the public, but they focus on new drugs and treatments that are backed by manufacturers with enough money to fund the necessary, expensive, multi-phased tests to get the FDA seal of approval.

The average out-of-pocket cost for obtaining a new drug approval is $802 million.[68] Unfortunately you can't get a patent on vitamin C or turmeric. Putting up that kind of capital to bring to market a substance that does not lend itself to market exclusivity, or the capacity to produce a return on investment, would be committing financial suicide.

As a result, instead of choosing prospective treatments because they work and are safe and easily accessible, the cancer industry puts billions of dollars in the opposite direction—developing drugs that have side effects, are capable of being proprietary, and, most importantly, can be sold for lots of money.

Unfortunately, with these rules and the focus on manufactured treatments, the FDA overlooks a whole class of natural therapies without the prospects of patents or profits and no sponsors to conduct the necessary tests to pass FDA hurdles. These include common herbs found in every kitchen spice rack that countless millennia of human experience suggest can be used to mitigate, prevent, and in some cases, cure disease.

What these home remedies can't hope to attain is the kind of FDA approval given to brand-name pharmaceuticals that would guarantee them a place among standard therapies doctors prescribe. As a result, many of these therapies get overlooked in the fight to kill cancer, and patients are left with only highly toxic chemicals for their treatment.

Some research into natural remedies is still going on and ironically even being funded in a few cases by the very same companies producing the synthetic cancer drugs. The government Biomedical and Life Sciences Database known as Medline (www.Medline.com) contains more than 21 million published study citations. While 2.6 million of them contain references to cancer treatment, 612 natural substances of potential value have been tested in a few thousand research studies.

13 Recognized Non-drug Super Supplements

There are more super supplements than what is on this list, but these were some of the best supplements researched for their cancer-fighting benefits.

If you're going to follow the "Don't Get It" plan, the key is to pick and choose which supplements you want to take, but at a minimum, begin with the first three. If you're currently diagnosed with cancer you'll need to take a lot more than these three and will definitely need a much higher dosage. That's why it's essential to work with a qualified doctor or clinic.

1. **VITAMIN D:** Vitamin D acts more like a hormone than a vitamin. Like a hormone, it has a huge impact on how genes express or fail to express themselves. In fact, one in every twenty-five genes in the human body interacts with vitamin D. This means that deficiencies may weaken the genetic infrastructure of our body.

Without vitamin D our immune system is incapable of producing certain antimicrobial substances, leaving our body unable to fight off bacteria, viruses, or cancer. A vitamin D deficiency will prevent the body from killing off precancerous cells before they turn into full-fledged cancer.

According to the Vitamin D Council, the human body needs from 3,000 to 5,000 IU daily, but current U.S. guidelines only recommend 600 IU a day for most adults and children. The daily dosage only rises at age seventy when the U.S. Institute of Medicine raises the recommendation to 800 IU.

2. **2-TO-1 RATIO OMEGA-6 TO OMEGA-3 FATTY ACIDS:** Greater intake of omega-3s has been associated with a reduced risk for cancer. By helping to stabilize the immune system and reducing the growth-promoting inflammatory cascade within the cancer cells themselves, omega-3s may have multiple anticancer effects, including regulating cell proliferation, inducing damaged cells to die, preventing blood vessel growth in tumors, and helping to prevent the spread of cancer cells to other parts of the body.

3. **VITAMIN C:** An indispensable factor in immune function, vitamin C enables our bodies to fight cancer naturally. Unlike most other mammals, we do not have the ability to produce this vitamin from glucose. We survive only because we obtain it from food, but many of us are literally dying slowly of scurvy (vitamin C deficiency). Our bodies produce hydrogen peroxide from vitamin C, if adequate quantities are provided, enabling our immune system to oxidize (burn) cancer cells. Due to the fact that the body may only absorb a certain amount, the remainder being excreted through the bowel in the well-known "bowel tolerance" laxative effect, it may be

necessary to use intravenous vitamin C therapy, by which far higher blood levels of vitamin C can be obtained.

4. CURCUMIN: Found in turmeric, curcumin displays antitumor and antioxidant properties. It reportedly inhibits cancer development by inducing apoptosis, or cell death in the tumor, without harming nearby healthy cells. It has also shown both chemoprotective and chemosensitizing properties, which means that it will both enhance the positive cancer-killing effects of conventional chemotherapy, and protect healthy cells which may be susceptible to being harmed by chemotherapy. Finally, it has an exceptionally high margin of safety, at least an order of magnitude greater than commonly used conventional chemotherapy agents such as 5-fluorouracil.

5. QUERCETIN: This plant-derived flavonoid is found in a wide range of fruits, vegetables and grains, and may be a major factor behind the well-known chemopreventive properties of these foods. A rather broad body of research shows that it induces programmed cell death in cancer cells. Other experimentally demonstrated anticancer properties include inducing cancer cell cycle arrest, sensitizing chemotherapy agents (making them more effective—chemosensitizer), and inhibiting tumor expansion (anti-angiogenic), to name but a few.[69]

6. ARTEMISIA: Also known as wormwood, artemisia is being researched as a safe, nontoxic, and inexpensive alternative for cancer patients. Research published in the Journal of Cancer Research and Clinical Oncology in 2010 indicates that the compound in wormwood known as dihydroartemisinin (DHA) could be developed as a novel agent against pancreatic cancer.[70]

7. COENZYME Q10 (COQ10): A naturally occurring enzyme in the body, CoQ10 is the catalyst of all cellular energy in the body. As cancer cells are developing, CoQ10 initiates apoptosis (self-destruction) of the cancer cells. CoQ10 is one of the most powerful antioxidants and protects the cells from damage by oxygen and stimulates immune function. It has been shown that cancer patients lack this vital enzyme in their blood. CoQ10 has been proven to inhibit oxidation, stimulate the immune system, and induce tumor remission. Deficiencies in CoQ10 have been documented in cancer patients. The ideal form is known as ubiquinol, which is a far more bioavailable and effective form of CoQ10.

8. PROBIOTICS: These friendly bacteria can decrease fecal enzymes associated with the formation of cancer-causing compounds in the intestines. They can bind to substances that cause genetic mutations to intestinal cells, and they stimulate enzymes that deactivate cancer-causing substances. Probiotics can also help support and stimulate the immune system indirectly and directly throughout the body, which is why they've been linked to a reduced risk for cancer.

9. RESVERATROL: Resveratrol is found in grapes, peanuts and plants, such as Japanese knotweed. One of its most documented properties is as an antioxidant. Antioxidants are responsible for putting out of commission the inflammatory, cell-damaging and ultimately DNA-damaging effects of excessive free radicals, which are molecules, atoms or ions that are highly chemically reactive. This may explain why resveratrol has been shown to slow aging and combat a wide range of cancers such as breast cancer, liver cancer, prostate cancer and colon cancer, to name but a few. While red wine and peanuts contain measurable quantities, it would take hundreds of bottles of wine and hundreds of pounds of peanuts to obtain what would be considered a therapeutic dose of resveratrol, somewhere between 200 and 500 milligrams daily, so for this you need to take a supplement.

10. GREEN TEA: An extract of the main active ingredient in green tea, EGCG, slows blood vessel formation in tumors, reducing the rate at which they can grow and spread. Green tea extract can also regulate cell division and growth and cause programmed cell death in DNA damaged cells.[71]

11. WHEATGRASS: Wheatgrass contains at least thirteen vitamins (several are antioxidants), including B12; many minerals and trace elements, including selenium; and all twenty amino acids. It also contains the hormone abscisic acid, antioxidant enzyme superoxide dismutase (SOD), and over thirty other enzymes, the antioxidant enzyme cytochrome oxidase, laetrile, and a whole lot of other nutrients. Wheatgrass, being such a potent source of many vitamins, minerals and plant enzymes, is said to be nature's own nutritional program. Wheatgrass also contains chlorophyll, which has almost the same molecular structure as hemoglobin. Chlorophyll increases hemoglobin production, meaning more oxygen gets to the cancer. Chlorophyll and selenium also help build the immunity system. Finally, wheatgrass is one of the most alkaline foods known to mankind (alkaline is the opposite of acid—cancer loves acid and hates alkaline). Wheatgrass can be taken fresh, or dehydrated wheatgrass is available in many greens products.

12. POLYMVA An acronym for polynucleotide reductase mineral, vitamins, and amino acids, this is a nontoxic antioxidant liquid formula composed of alpha lipoic acid and the element palladium. Among the vitamins it contains are B12 and others of the B complex. It's promoted as a nutritional supplement that is a nontoxic alternative to chemotherapy. Because it's said to be able to cross the blood-brain barrier, this product is usually used with brain tumors, but it's also said to be effective against tumors in the lung, ovaries, and breast. It's also thought to boost the immune system, reduce pain, and help people regain energy and appetite. It's considered a powerful antioxidant that can turn the toxins released by cancer into energy. According to its manufacturers, the compound attacks cancerous cells and protects DNA and RNA. They contend that the lipoic acid allows the various minerals, vitamins, and amino acids to be easily absorbed into the system where they can kill cancerous cells. You can call 800-960-6760 for a packet of info or to order the product, or go to the website (www.polymva.net).

13. SELENIUM: This is an exceptionally important mineral without which our cells can't adequately detoxify and protect themselves against free radical damage, two things that can contribute to cancer. Without it, our thyroid can't function, and our cells can't produce glutathione, an essential enzyme in both protecting against T-cellular oxidative damage which may lead to cancer, as well as directly inducing death in the cancer cells themselves.

Because modern soils do not contain selenium and plants don't need it to grow, the mineral is rarely found in the modern diet. It only takes one-fifth of a milligram a day to prevent a clinical deficiency, which is infinitesimal relative to the weight of our bodies. It's also crucially important that you take the appropriate form of selenium. Most mass-market supplements, for instance, use either sodium selenite or sodium selenate, both in forms that can be highly toxic. The form most suitable for cancer prevention is yeast-grown selenomethionine or an organically-bound source such as Brazil nuts.

Selenium, in many ways, exemplifies how important even the smallest component of our bodily system is to the health of the whole.

TOP 10 NONTOXIC THERAPY PROGRAMS

1. The Budwig Protocol

Dr. Johanna Budwig was a German biochemist and a seven-time Nobel nominee. She discovered that our diets often lack highly unsaturated fatty acids and contain an excess of manmade oils known as trans fats (or partially hydrogenated oils).

These trans fats are "bad fats" found in most of the cooking oils sold in grocery stores and used in lots of products, including almost all fast foods. Most of these oils are derived from corn, sunflowers, and other plants by using extreme heat and chemicals. They have a twenty-year shelf life and, when ingested, destroy the electrical charge in our cell membranes. Without the charge, our cells don't get enough oxygen and start to suffocate. (Remember, cancer is anaerobic.) When our cells suffocate and are deprived of their proper electrical field, we become more susceptible to chronic and terminal diseases.

Dr. Budwig's research also demonstrated that the lack of essential unsaturated fats is responsible for the production of oxidase, which induces cancer growth and causes many other chronic disorders. She came to the understanding that cancer was not the result of too much cell growth, but defective cell growth, caused by too many bad fats and not enough healthy fats.

Good health requires the proper ratio of 2:1, Omega-6 to Omega-3. Dr. Budwig believed that cancer and chronic disease are the result of this ratio being thrown out of balance by the ingestion of too many bad fats. When this ratio is off, oxygen can't be pulled into the cell, which is necessary for healthy, normal cells. Cancer cells thrive on this absence of oxygen, so restoring oxygen to these cells is a crucial first step to restoring health.

The Budwig protocol is based on a determination that healthy fats must first be bound to a sulfur-based protein before being consumed. That allows them to become water-soluble, which in turn permits their penetration into the cell.

HERE IS THE PROTOCOL:

Only use flax oil from the refrigerated section of your health food store. Never use capsules, flakes, or flax oil from the shelves. It must be refrigerated. And check the expiration date to make sure it hasn't expired. The mixing ratio is two tablespoons of cottage cheese to one tablespoon of oil. Mix only the amount you're consuming at one time so it's mixed fresh each and every time.

One example would be to mix four tablespoons of cottage cheese with two tablespoons of flax oil. This should be consumed twice daily, or more depending on the severity of the health condition one is attempting to address. One should probably start slowly with the oil, maybe just once a day and work their way up letting the body adjust to the protocol.

The oil and the cottage cheese must be thoroughly mixed at a low speed, using an immersion blender. It should be mixed until a creamy texture is achieved, with no standing oil. Let stand for a few minutes, then consume immediately. Do not add anything to the mixture until after it's mixed and left standing for a few minutes. At this time you can add stevia and berries to improve the taste.

The protocol is made even more effective by sprinkling a tablespoon or two of freshly ground flax seed over the freshly mixed flax oil and cottage cheese mixture. Mix this in by hand. This supercharges the protocol. Do not buy pre-ground flax seed, as the flax seed goes rancid fifteen minutes after grinding.

2. Proteolytic Enzyme Therapy

There are two theories about how proteolytic enzymes work. The first was developed by John Beard, a doctor in Wales, at the turn of the last century. Dr. Beard discovered that pancreatic enzymes destroy cancer cells. One of his most brilliant observations was that the fetal pancreas starts working and secreting enzymes at the 56th day of gestation. Given that fetuses don't digest anything until they're born, Beard wondered why the pancreas started producing enzymes so early. He noticed that the day the pancreas started producing enzymes was the day the placenta stopped growing. His theory was that many placental cells remain in our body. When these misplaced placental cells get lost, they can start growing and turn cancerous if you don't have enough pancreatic enzymes to shut them off. (By the way, the medical community for a long time thought Dr. Beard was crazy. Now, a hundred years later, technology has confirmed that these cells do persist in our bodies.)

The second theory, based on research findings, contends that high doses of pancreatic enzymes can destroy an outer layer of protective protein coating on cancer cells, making them more vulnerable to immune system defenses. Most alternative doctors who operate under this theory will combine other treatments with the pancreatic enzymes, which will enhance their cancer-killing ability. Other benefits of these enzymes include decreasing inflammation and increasing the macrophages and killer cells.

3. I.V. Vitamin C Therapy

In the 1970s Hugh D. Riordan, M.D. and his colleagues researched and implemented vitamin C therapy as an adjuvant to conventional cancer treatment. He noted in his research that patients with cancer were generally deficient in ascorbic acid and therefore had a reduced ability to induce tumor cytotoxicity, which is essentially cell death.

It was also clear that taking vitamin C orally, even in megadoses, did not increase its concentration in the blood sufficiently to initiate this cell destruction. For this reason, Riordan and his colleagues turned to intravenous administration of ascorbic acid.

Indeed, Riordan's work led other oncologists to experiment with Vitamin C in their practices. One such oncologist, Victor Marcial, M.D., gave patients with advanced stage cancer between 40,000 and 75,000 milligrams intravenously several times a week. He reported that in the initial stages of the treatment 75% of his patients experienced a reduction in tumor size of at least 50 percent. "As a radiation oncologist, I also give radiation therapy," Riordan said. "Vitamin C has two effects. It increases the beneficial effects of radiation and chemotherapy and decreases the adverse effects. But this is not a subtle effect, not 15 or 20%. It's a dramatic effect. Once you start using IV vitamin C, the effect is so dramatic that it's difficult to go back to not using it."[72 73 74]

One of the fascinating paradoxes of vitamin C and cancer is that cancer cells are known to contain relatively high amounts of it, often depleting the surrounding healthy tissues and blood of vitamin C in order to attain these elevated quantities. Glucose, a preferred fuel source of cancer cells, is actually only four metabolic steps away from vitamin C. It's possible that cancer cells mistake vitamin C for Glucose and absorb it in high amounts as a result. Either way, when large amounts of vitamin C are injected into the blood, it accumulates in the cancer cells in unusually high amounts. It then behaves as a pro-oxidant as it interacts with intracellular copper and iron. This cellular biochemical reaction produces hydrogen peroxide as a result, which can oxidize and kill cancerous cells with relatively low collateral damage to healthy tissue. In fact, hydrogen peroxide is one of the chemicals our white blood cells use to kill pathogens and cancerous cells.

4. I.V. Ozone Treatment

Ozone (O3) is a highly active form of oxygen. This therapy brings elevated concentrations of oxygen into the blood stream. In this therapy, blood is taken out of the patient, oxygenated, then put directly back into the body. At this point the new blood is fully oxygenated causing a lot of beneficial effects. The most important is replenishing oxygen to the body quickly. Nobel Prize winner Dr. Otto Warburg showed that cancer cells do not occur in a healthy, oxygenated environment. Many think the lack of oxygen is the prime cause of all cancers. Flooding the cells with oxygen slows the growth of cancer cells and even helps them to return to normal. Another benefit is cleansing the blood of viruses and bacteria.

5. Hyperthermia

Raising the body temperature induces an artificial fever, thereby increasing blood flow and oxygenating the body. This boosts the immune system and helps detoxify the body, just like a normal fever does during a sickness. Unlike normal cells, cancer cells can't tolerate heat, and many die. The principle is the same as a fever. Our immune system gives us a fever for the purpose of fighting an infection because the high temperatures kill the microbes, viruses, and bacteria while leaving our own cells undamaged.

The typical hyperthermia treatment can take up to five hours. During the first two hours the patient's body temperature is gradually raised to about 105 degrees Fahrenheit. This temperature is maintained for two hours, and then over the next two hours the patient's body temperature is brought back down to normal. A doctor is carefully monitoring the patient's vital signs also makes sure that the patient's hydration is replenished and maintained the whole time. This is how hyperthermia is able to kill millions of cancer cells. Any cancer cells that remain are now weaker, enabling another therapy that raises the immune system to kill them off.

6. Coffee Enemas

When a coffee enema is used, the caffeine from the coffee is absorbed and goes directly to the liver where it becomes a very strong detoxifier by causing the liver to produce more bile. That in turn moves toxins out toward the small intestine for elimination. This frees up the liver to help process more incoming toxic materials that have accumulated in the organs, tissues and bloodstream and eliminate them as well. The coffee contains some alkaloids that also stimulate the production of glutathione-S-transferase, an enzyme used by the liver to make the detox pathways run.

Boil one quart of water in a non-aluminum pot. Add two tablespoons or more of coffee and continue to boil for five minutes. Remove pot from the heat and add one tablespoon of unsulfured molasses (optional). Cool to 90 degrees Fahrenheit or less. Pour the coffee mixture through a fine mesh strainer into two one-cup measuring cups. Clamp the end of the enema bag. Pour one cup of filtered coffee mixture into the enema bag. To clear the line of air, release the clamp until the coffee begins to flow out. Then clamp the bag again immediately.

Hang the enema bag at a height of about three feet, not higher. Lie on the floor and gently insert the nozzle. Use olive oil on the nozzle if needed. Release the clamp and let the coffee mixture flow into the sigmoid colon. Clamp the tubing as soon as there is a sensation of "fullness" or when the enema bag is empty, and remove the nozzle. If possible, without forcing yourself, retain the enema for ten minutes. Then empty your bowel.

After emptying your bowel, repeat the process with the remaining (one cup) of coffee mixture. If you can't hold one cup of coffee mixture enema, take several smaller enemas, and you do not need to reheat the coffee.

When the bile duct empties, you'll hear or feel a squirting sensation in the area of your right rib cage. After feeling the bile emptying, you can stop taking enemas for that day.

If you do not feel the bile duct emptying after one week of daily enemas, increase the strength of the coffee or take slightly larger volume enemas. If you feel you are emptying bile duct, you will not need to do a second enema or increase the volume.

You should not feel nervous or jittery after the enema because the coffee does not get absorbed systemically. If you do feel nervous, jittery, have palpitations, or irregular heartbeats after a coffee enema, reduce the amount of coffee by half or more.

Repeat enemas as needed to detoxify chemical toxins and/or allergic reactions.

7. Ultraviolet Blood Irradiation Therapy (UVBI)

UVBI Therapy produces similar effects as Ozone Blood Therapy. In this therapy, a portion of the patient's blood is removed, then exposed to UVC light before being put back into body. The effects of this therapy are:

• Improved circulation and oxygenation of tissues.

• Decreased inflammation.

• Powerful anti-infection ability that is known to kill ongoing viruses.

• Stimulation of the immune system.

8. I.V. Hydrogen Peroxide

This is a type of ozone treatment. Hydrogen peroxide (H2O2) is super abundant in oxygen. When administered intravenously it supplies this wealth of oxygen to the cancer cells. Since cancer thrives in an anaerobic state and does not do well in the presence of oxygen, the effect is to inhibit or destroy the cancer.

9. Juicing

You need to look at juicing in the same way a doctor would look at IV therapy for a patient, even though we're talking about taking the juices orally. It's something that can go right into your bloodstream and flood the body with vitamins, nutrients, and minerals. This is why we put this in the category of therapies instead of supplements.

Juicing is extremely important for two reasons. First, it helps the vitamins and minerals in vegetables or fruit to be digested much more quickly and easily because you have eliminated all the fiber from it. Second, you can consume ten to a hundred times more vegetables or fruits in juices than if you were to eat them whole.

The next question we always get is, "What are the best vegetables and fruits to juice?" We don't recommend juicing fruits, even though fruits have some amazing nutrients. They are sugar and when juiced they spike insulin levels very high, very quickly. So if you're to do any fruits, make sure it's a small amount, and stick to your lowest glycemic fruits like green apples as well as most berries. Also, inside of the apple are the apple seeds which are powerful in killing cancer, so make sure that if you juice apples, you use the whole apple, including the seeds.

TOP VEGETABLES TO JUICE:

1. Broccoli
2. Green asparagus
3. Kale
4. Cabbage
5. Cauliflower
6. Peppers
7. Spinach
8. Red beets (beetroot)
9. Swiss chard
10. Carrots

HERE ARE JUST A FEW OF THE CANCER CELL-KILLING NUTRIENTS (DIRECT OR INDIRECT) IN VEGETABLES:

- Sulforaphanes/isothiocyanates in raw broccoli

- Isothiocyanates in raw cabbage

- Saponins in green asparagus

- Proanthocyanidins in beetroot/red beets

Carrots raise blood sugar levels, but the reason why we still include them in the top ten is because of all the beneficial nutrients carrots have. As in virtually all vegetables, there are hundreds, if not thousands, of phytonutrients in carrots that have not yet been identified or tested for cancer-fighting abilities. But based on many testimonials, carrots may be the best cancer-fighting vegetable of all. They're full of alpha carotene, beta carotene, vitamin E, and much more. This is why we always add two or three carrots every time we juice, and hundreds of cancer patients who only juice carrots have amazing results. Again, be careful of the high Insulin reaction.

10. Hyperbaric Oxygen Therapy (HBOT)

HBOT delivers 100% pure oxygen to you through increased atmospheric pressure in an enclosed chamber. When oxygen is delivered at higher than normal pressure, your body is able to absorb more of it into your blood cells, blood plasma, cerebral-spinal fluid, and other bodily fluids.

Once in the chamber, your body responds by reducing inflammation, which in turn increases blood flow to oxygen-deprived areas.

HYPERBARIC OXYGEN THERAPY ALSO:

- Saturates your body with oxygen (including the Plasma and White Cells).

- Increases your oxygen level by 20 to 30 percent.

- Increases your ability to fight infections.

- Creates new capillaries and increases blood flow.

- Clears and deactivates toxins and metabolic waste.

- Stimulates your body to create new blood cells.

- Increases your stem cell production 800% (after forty treatments).

- Accelerates your rate of healing.

CHAPTER 14
TOP SUPPLEMENTS THAT BOOST THE Immune System

One of the keys to being a Cancer Killer is to have a strong immune system. Here is a list of supplements that help raise the immune system. Pick one of these to add to your "Don't Get It" plan.

1. MEDICINAL MUSHROOMS: Choose maiitake, reishi or shiitake mushrooms. The amazing thing about these three mushrooms is that they're foods and medicines, simultaneously nourishing the body while increasing immune function. Mushrooms, in particular, boost the functionality of the natural killer cells, part of the innate immune system. They're hugely important in tumor immune-surveillance because they're capable of directly killing tumor cells.

2. AHCC: This stands for Active Hexose Correlated Compound, and is classified as a functional food made from hybridized mycelia of shiitake (and sometimes other mushrooms) in rice bran. It contains both alpha and beta-glucan polysaccharides, well-known modulators of immunity. What is so unique about this compound is that it's an anticancer agent, controlled by your body, that combats cancer by boosting your immune function. This is a radically different approach versus conventional chemotherapy, which poisons rapidly dividing cells, indiscriminately killing both cancer and immune cells (among other healthy cell types).

3. BETA-1,3-D-GLUCAN: This compound is found in the cellulose in most plants, the bran of cereal grains, and in mushrooms, fungi, yeast and bacteria. It's known as a biological-response modifier for its ability to activate the immune system. Interestingly, it's able to regulate an immune system that is either overactive or suppressed. A shiitake derived beta-glucan extract known as lentian has been specifically studied for its ability to boost the anticancer effects of chemotherapy agents, and produce significantly longer survival times in cancer patients.[75]

4. IP6: Known as Inositol Hexaphosphate (IP6) or phytate when in salt form, it is especially prevalent in the bran and seeds of plants. It's rich in phosphorous. It's classified as an anti-nutrient because it binds with certain minerals and vitamins, reducing their absorption. But this chelating mechanism is also behind its anticancer properties. For instance, it's capable of depleting iron within the body, which is an essential factor in the rapid reproduction of certain cancer cells. A metabolite of IP6 known as InsP1-5 is in fact found within most mammalian cells, where it's believed to play an important role in regulating the vital functions of the cells. One study published in 1995 in the Journal of Nutrition found that InsP6 was able not only to suppress the growth of cancer cells, but was able to regress malignant T-cells back to a normal phenotype by enhancing its differentiation.[76]

5. MGN-3: This is actually an extract of rice bran enzymatically treated with extracts of mushrooms like shiitake. It has been shown to increase natural killer cell activity up to 300%, enabling the body to launch a direct attack on cancer and precancerous cells.

DR. MAJORS' STORY: DOCTOR, HEAL THYSELF

Overcoming Cancer and Getting Back to Living

We arrived in Reno on Thursday evening and checked into a hotel. Although I was exhausted from the trip, I felt a new sense of purpose. I felt confident that Dr. Forsythe would get to the root of my cancer. I felt confident. First thing on Friday morning, after a restless night for both my wife and me, we headed to see the man who would help me turn my health around. I was Dr. Forsythe's first patient of the day. His exterior is very placid, almost gentle. What struck me was how much hope he exuded. Without cutting me open, burning me, or poisoning me with high doses of chemotherapy, he was confident he could get my cancer under control.

But while his demeanor was kind and unruffled, he made it clear we had no time to procrastinate. Immediately, they began tests to find out what caused my cancer. One of the first tests he did was the Greek blood test, for which they literally whisked off on a plane to Greece that afternoon. There, the researchers would extract the cancer cells from my blood and then subject them to tests involving twenty different supplements to see which would be the most effective on my cancer.

The results would not be back for almost three weeks. Until then, Dr. Forsythe would start me on protocols he had used successfully before on the same type of cancer. He began with intravenous (IV) Vitamin C; IV hydrogen peroxide to infuse my body with more oxygen; IV PolyMVA; and his own Forsythe Formula for maximum nutrition.

I was also working closely with a Homeopath and Nutritionist, meeting with them several times a day. I continued this protocol for about three weeks, while my wife and I lived in a nearby hotel. Finally, the results of the Greek blood test came back, and they began giving me the exact supplements the test showed killed my cancer. I also had done specific toxicity testing to see the exact toxins in my bloodstream.

Although still weak, I knew I had to begin getting some exercise to help replenish my body with oxygen. My wife would help me get on a stationary bike, and I would begin peddling for about ten seconds, then rest for about thirty seconds. Each day I would increase that as my stamina began to return. Soon I was able to lift some small weights. I continued doing the surge workouts, which I knew was the quickest and best way to build muscle and bring oxygen into my body. Short duration, high intensity Surge/Max T3 workouts daily.

After three weeks, it was finally time to fly home. Just to see my children again after believing for a while I would not, gave me new energy and commitment. I was feeling better, but I still had a long way to go. The next step was an intense detoxification, removing as many toxins as possible while I prepared to begin a rigorous schedule of very precise eating and supplements. I was taking about ten times the normal dosage, depending on the supplement. Dosages like this can be dangerous, which is why it's crucial to work with someone who knows what they're doing.

Every cancer is different, and every person is different. There's not a one-size-fits-all approach to cancer, so having a trusted alternative cancer center to work with is vital. Some people will eat completely raw and get better; some will eat meat and get better. Some cancers are caused by too much acidity, so the patient must follow an alkaline diet. But if a cancer is alkaline, a more alkaline diet will make the person sicker.

The most important thing I had to do was cut out all sugar of any type. That meant no grains, no pasta, and no fruit of any kind. Sugar is fuel for cancer, and it was time to cut this cancer off. I followed what I now call the advanced cancer eating plan, which is 70% carbs from vegetables, 20% good healthy fats, and 10% good protein from only organic turkey and chicken and organic, grass-fed red meat.

Again, this was my protocol. It's what I believed I needed based on the information I had about my cancer. I knew there wasn't just one cause for cancer. I wanted to follow the Five Essentials, so the protocols I chose were based on those five—mindset, central nervous system, nutrition, oxygen, and toxicity.

First, I needed to cleanse. Here is the order of detoxification:

1. Bowel/colon cleanse (three colonics is best).

2. Viral cleanse.

3. Parasite cleanse.

4. Fungal cleanse.

5. Blood cleanse.

6. Dental cleanup: root canals (which are an ongoing bacterial infection), amalgam, cavitations (pockets inside jaw bone left after extraction of wisdom and molar teeth which holds bacteria).

7. Kidney cleanse.

8. Liver cleanse/gallbladder cleanse (liver flush).

Once the liver had been cleansed, I was ready for coffee enemas twice a day. (You can do more than that depending on your case.)

6:00 A.M.:	Two tablespoons of greens (made up of alfalfa, barley, and wheat grass).
6:05 A.M.:	15 minute short duration, high intensity workout.
6:30 A.M.:	Twenty pancreatic enzymes on empty stomach (one hour away from food).
7:30 A.M.:	Power-food protein smoothie (2 tablespoons of power-food, 1 scoop of grass-fed/hormone free protein, handful of kale or leafy greens, 2 cups of almond milk).
7:30 A.M.:	Morning Supplements: PolyMVA, quercitin, 5000 IU of vitamin D, 5000 mg of vitamin C, CoQ10, curcumin, artemisia, took variety of mushrooms that raise immune system, 2-to-1 ratio omegas).
8:00 A.M.:	100 billion units of Probiotics.
9:30 A.M.:	20 pancreatic enzymes.
10:00 A.M.:	Drank Budwig protocol.
11:15 A.M.:	8 ounces juice (kale, cabbage, broccoli, carrot, beetroot, spinach, Swiss chard).
12:00 P.M.:	Lunch (salad with organic chicken or turkey, olive oil and vegetables).
12:00 P.M.:	Afternoon supplements: PolyMVA, Quercitin, CoQ10, curcumin, artemisia, cordychi and MyCommunity (two varieties of mushrooms that raise Immune System).
2:00 P.M.:	Twenty Pancreatic enzymes.
6:00 P.M.:	Juice (same as earlier juice).
6:15 P.M.:	Dinner (organic chicken or turkey or organic, grass-fed red meat with side of vegetables; a lot of my meals were made from Advanced Plan recipes).
7:00 P.M.:	Drank Budwig protocol.
8:00 P.M.:	Twenty pancreatic enzymes.
9:00 P.M.:	Power-food protein smoothie (2 tablespoons of powerfood, 1 scoop of grass-fed/hormone free protein, handful of kale or leafy green, 2 cups of almond milk, and raw cacao).
9:00 P.M.:	Night supplements: PolyMVA, Quercetin, 5000 IU of Vitamin D, 5000 mg of Vitamin C, CoQ10, curcumin, artemisia, cordychi and Mycommunity (two varieties of medicinal mushrooms that raise immune system).

Slept at least nine hours a night for ultimate repair and growth.

You need to cycle off your supplements about every four weeks. Take five days off from taking your supplements to give your liver a rest. The days you're off your supplements can be just as important as the days you're taking them. Continue doing coffee enemas daily. You need to be drinking at least eight cups of clean-filtered or toxin-free water a day, away from meals, in addition to the juices and teas. Don't drink when you eat, either. Meat is tough on the body because it takes so much energy to digest it, so I rarely ate meat at dinner time; breakfast and lunch are the best times to eat meat.

I also had X-rays of my spine taken and sent to Dr. Tony Nalda, one of the best corrective care chiropractors in the world. He found major upper cervical damage, loss of my cervical curve, damaged ligaments, and a slight curvature in my lower back. He gave me recommendations on how I needed to be adjusted to remove subluxations and allow my brain to have 100% communication with my body so it could heal. I was adjusted at least three times per week for three months. I was also doing my at-home spinal corrective exercises two times per day for three months. At that point my new X-rays were much better, and I knew the cancer had to be gone! I continued from there being adjusted three times a week.

Every day I would also go into an infrared sauna at over 140 degrees, which would help detoxify my body as well as make my cancer weaker and more susceptible to dying. I would wake up each morning doing a tapping (EFT) technique to release any negative emotions that I was still holding on to. This was my normal daily routine for months until I went to Spain.

In February 2011, I headed for Spain with three colleagues to a clinic run by Dr. Raymond Hilu in the seaside town of Malaga. A specialist in treating late-stage disease, Dr. Hilu had studied under renowned cancer specialist Johanna Budwig.

Dr. Hilu is the head of the Foundation for Alternative and Integrative Medicine, a medical organization that searches the world for effective, nontoxic, and low-cost alternative medical therapies. Dr. Hilu employed techniques not available in the U.S., such as using ozone to clean the blood and help replenish its oxygen.

When I got to Dr. Hilu's clinic, he used blood microscopy, which is analysis of blood by means of a high-powered microscope that can magnify cells to twenty-five thousand times their normal size. Although I was feeling better, my blood was still toxic. I needed to begin detox protocols right away or risk the return of my cancer.

I began with three colonics to make sure my colon was clean and then had three flax oil enemas, which enables the flax oil to absorb quickly into the bloodstream. As they were detoxifying me, I began doing ozone blood cleaning, Papimi (an electromagnetic energy device where a high voltage is passed as a magnetic field through the body, penetrating every tissue), and different oxygen therapies.

I was prepared to stay in Spain until my blood was clear and I was back to normal. As it turned out, Dr. Hilu only needed two weeks.

When I got home, I continued the Advanced, no grain or sugar, cancer eating plan as well as all of my supplements, infrared sauna, specific chiropractic adjustments three times a week, and surge workouts (high intensity/short duration workouts) six days a week. I woke up every day doing my EFT/tapping protocol. I was also going to Contemporary Medicine in Burr Ridge, Illinois every two weeks where Dr. Ather Malik and Dr. Thomas Hesselink did IV vitamin C, IV H2O2 (hydrogen peroxide), and UV blood cleaning. I will continue to go there getting blood work every three to four months and IVs for at least five years! Cancer has a memory, and any time I let my guard down, it has an opportunity to come back. Staying one step ahead lets me be a Cancer Killer all the time! (I do not follow Budwig protocol when doing high amounts of vitamin C, because this can offset the beneficial effects of the Budwig).

I also had one dead tooth that was full of bacteria, and cavitations from four molars pulled years ago that were full of bacteria. All of that had to be addressed to stop the bacteria dripping into my bloodstream and weakening my immune system. I went to Dr. Paul Gallo, DDS, who is one of the top holistic dentists in the world and follows the proper protocols to remove a dead tooth and clean up all the bacteria left behind.

While none of this was easy, I want to make it clear it wasn't a fight either. I wasn't in a battle with cancer. I was getting myself healthy and never stopping! I also do blood work every three to four months to monitor tumor markers, vitamin D, and my iron levels. I will continue this protocol for another five years, then gradually decrease it. If I see that my blood work gets worse or tumor markers go up, I will immediately stop everything and fly to Spain, Nevada, or South Carolina where Dr. Dalal Akoury, an oncologist who specializes in alternative oncology, reviews my blood work regularly.

It hasn't been an easy two years since my first headaches. I have been on a journey of discovery about my body with my friends and family. And it's far from over. Yet, at a time when many would choose to grieve the discovery of cancer, I have chosen to study it. At a time when many would choose to put their lives on hold, my wife and I had our fourth child. This isn't a trite tale that culminates in self-help platitudes about turning lemons into lemonade. I was facing life or death. I chose not to follow the medical establishment down a road of pain and poison. Instead I chose to cleanse my body and life of toxins and stress and immerse myself in the positive and natural. I chose to get to the cause, get myself healthy, become a Cancer Killer, and live!

Alternative Cancer Clinics

Before I counsel anyone to call or visit one of these alternative cancer clinics, I make sure I prepare them for what may occur. You have to realize that most of these doctors have left traditional medicine. Right away you know, "they must be different," but different in an amazing way. They're very, very busy, so they get disorganized and don't return calls right away. Please bear with them! When you're dealing with cancer, you're experiencing such fear. Every second feels like hours. You want answers now and want to be taken care of now, and sometimes that isn't possible. Just remember all of that when you think about heading to an alternative treatment facility.

Your health insurance will pay $200,000 or more for a cancer patient to use traditional medical treatments (cutting, burning, poisoning) but is likely to deny coverage for the $10,000 to $50,000 for an alternative cancer treatment, which is more effective!

Here is a brief list of clinics in and out of the U.S. and Canada in no particular order. Do your own research to figure out where you want to go and where you feel comfortable. There are many clinics. Talk to them and talk to others that have used them. Then it's up to you. Decide which one is best for you. Many of them can give you more artillery in your efforts to become a Cancer Killer.

CENTURY WELLNESS CLINIC
Dr. James Forsysthe
Reno, Nevada
1.877.789.0707 (toll free)
www.centurywellness.com

**FOUNDATION FOR ALTERNATIVE
AND INTEGRATIVE MEDICINE**
Dr. Raymond Hilu
Marbella, Spain
952 90 77 77
www.institutohilu.com

CONTEMPORARY MEDICINE
Dr. Ather A. Malik & Dr. Thomas L. Hesselink
Burr Ridge, Illinois
630.321.9010
www.contemporarymedicine.net

DR. NICHOLAS GONZALEZ
New York City
212.213.3337
www.dr-gonzalez.com

OASIS OF HOPE
Tijuana, Mexico
1.888.500.4673 (toll free)
www.oasisofhope.com

THE NEVADA CENTER OF ALTERNATIVE AND ANTI-AGING MEDICINE
Carson City, Nevada
775.884.3990 (toll free)
www.antiagingmedicine.com

NEW HOPE MEDICAL CENTER
Scottsdale, Arizona
1.866.524.4673 (toll free)
www.newhopemedicalcenter.com

CLINIC OF BIOMEDICINE
Toronto, Ontario, Canada
1.855.705.3325 (toll free)
www.biomedici.ca

AN OASIS OF HEALING
Mesa, Arizona
480-834-5414
www.anoasisofhealing.com

CITATIONS

1. *Surveillance, Epidemiology, and End Results Program. Cancer Facts & the War on Cancer.* 2002.

2. Cancer Facts and Figures 2012, American Cancer Society Inc., Surveillance Research

3. "The Cost of Cancer," last modified February 18, 2011, National Cancer Institute, http://www.cancer.gov/aboutnci/servingpeople/cancer-statistics/costofcancer.

4. C B Hong, J M Winston, L P Thornburg, C C Lee, J S WSoods. Follow-up study on the carcinogenicity of vinyl chloride and vinylidene chloride in rats and mice: tumor incidence and mortality subsequent to exposure. *J Toxicol Environ Health.* 1981 Jun ;7(6):909-24.

5. Hong, C.B. and J. M. Winston, L. P. Thornburg, C. C. Lee, J. S. WSoods JS, "Follow-Up Study on the Carcinogenicity of Vinyl Chloride and Vinylidene Chloride in Rats and Mice: Tumor Incidence and Mortality Subsequent to Exposure," *Journal of Toxicology and Environmental Health*, June 1981, 7(6):909-24, PubMed, PMID:7265317, http://www.ncbi.nlm.nih.gov/pubmed/7265317.

6. PreventCancer.com, Mammography Awareness: Chemical Industry Funds Breast Cancer Campaign

7. Ji, Sayer. "How X-Ray Mammography Is Accelerating the Epidemic of Cancer," June 8, 2012. GreenMedInfo.com.

8. "Effect of Screening Mammography on Breast-cancer Mortality in Norway," *New England Journal of Medicine*, 2010 Sep 23 ;363(13):1203-10.

9. U.S. Preventive Services Task Force (USPSTF) Recommendations, Screening for Breast Cancer, Dec. 2009 Update

10. "Screening for breast cancer Recommendation Statement," U.S. Preventive Services Task Force, Updated December 2009, http://www.uspreventiveservicestaskforce.org/uspstf09/breastcancer/brcanrs.htm.

11. "Cancer Research Funding," National Cancer Institute, last modified June 2, 2011, http://www.cancer.gov/cancertopics/factsheet/NCI/research-funding.

12. Angela B Mariotto, K Robin Yabroff, Yongwu Shao, Eric J Feuer, Martin L Brown. Projections of the cost of cancer care in the United States: 2010-2020. J Natl Cancer Inst. 2011 Jan 19 ;103(2):117-28.

13. Morgan, G. and R. Ward, M. Barton, "The Contribution of Cytotoxic Chemotherapy to 5-year survival in adult malignancies," *Journal of Clinical Oncology*, December 2004, 16(8):549-60, PubMed, PMID:15630849.

14. "Ionizing Radiation and Tobacco Use Increases The Risk of a Subsequent Lung Carcinoma In Women With Breast Cancer," Case-Only Design. *The Journal of Clinical Oncology* 2005 Oct 20;23(30):7467-74.

15. "Table 16: Fruits and Vegetables and Breast Cancer Risk," Susan G. Komen for the Cure, updated July 7, 2011, http://ww5.komen.org/ContentNoSidebar. aspx?id=6030&terms=fruits%20and%20vegetables.

16. World Health Organization, Genes and Human Disease: http://www.who.int/ genomics/public/geneticdiseases/en/index2.html

17. Wang, Linda and Katherine Arnold, "Risk from breast cancer Susceptibility Gene May be Exaggerated in Most Studies," *Journal of the National Cancer Institute*, (2002) 94 (16): 1183, http://jnci.oxfordjournals.org/content/94/16/1183.3.full.

18. Ornish, Dean, and Mark Jesus M. Magbanua, Gerdi Weidner, Vivian Weinberg, Colleen Kemp, Christopher Green, Michael D. Mattie, Ruth Marlin, Jeff Simko, Katsuto Shinohara, Christopher M. Hagg, Peter R. Carroll, "Changes in Prostate Gene Expression in Men Undergoing an Intensive Nutrition and Lifestyle Invervention," Proceedings of the National Academy of Sciences, June 17, 2008, Vol. 105, No. 24, 8369-8374, www.pnas.org_cgi_ doi_10.1073_pnas.0803080105.

19. Associated Press, "Experts: One-third of breast cancer Cases Avoidable," USA Today, March 25, 2010, http://www.usatoday.com/news/health/2010-03-25-breast-cancer_N.htm.

20. Elenkov, I. J. and R. L. Wilder, G. P. Chrousos, E. S. Vizi, "The Sympathetic Nerve— An Integrative Interface Between Two Supersystems: The Brain and the Immune System," *Pharmacological Reviews*, December 2000, 52(4):595-638, PubMed, PMID:11121511, http://www.ncbi.nlm.nih.gov/pubmed/11121511.

21. Teodorczyk-Injeyan, Julita A. and Marion McGregor, Richard Ruegg, H. Stephen Injeyan, "Interleukin 2-Regulated In Vitro Antibody Production Following A Single Spinal Manipulative Treatment In Normal Subjects," *Chiropractic & Osteopathy*, September 8, 2010, 18:26, PubMed 20825650, http://www.ncbi.nlm.nih.gov/ pubmed/20825650.

22. Selano, J.L. and B. C. Hightower, B. Pfleger, K. Feeley-Collins, J. D. Grostic, "The Effects of Specific Upper Cervical Adjustments on the CD4 Counts of HIV Positive Patients," *Chiropractic Research Journal*, 1994, 3(1)

23. Takeda, Yasuhiko and Shouji Arai, "Relationship Between Vertebral Deformities And Allergic Diseases," *The Internet Journal of Orthopedic Surgery*, 2004 Volume 2 Number 1, Internet Scientific Publications, accessed June 21, 2012, http://www. ispub.com/journal/the-internet-journal-of-orthopedic-surgery/volume-2-number-1/ relationship-between-vertebral-deformities-and-allergic-diseases.html.

24. Epstein, Samuel S., "A Needless New Risk of breast cancer," *Los Angeles Times*, March 20, 1994, accessed June 21, 2012, http://articles.latimes. com/1994-03-20/opinion/op-36250_1_breast-cancer-risks.

25. LeRoith, D. and H. Werner, S. Neuenschwander, T. Kalebic, and L. J. Helman, (1995), "The Role of the Insulin-like Growth Factor-I Receptor in Cancer," *Annals of the New York Academy of Sciences*, 766: 402–408. doi: 10.1111/ j.1749-6632.1995.tb26689.x.

26. Mantzoros, C.S. and A. Tzonou, L. B. Signorello, M. Stampfer, D. Trichopoulos, H.O. Adami, "Insulin-Like Growth Factor 1 in Relation to Prostate Cancer and Benign Prostatic Hyperplasia," *British Journal of Cancer*, Vol. 76, No. 9, 1997, pp. 1115-18, PubMed, PMID:9365156.

27. Cascinu, S. and E. Del Ferro, C. Grianti, M. Ligi, R. Ghiselli, G. Foglietti, V. Saba, F. Lungarotti, G. Catalano, "Inhibition Of Tumor Cell Kinetics and Serum Insulin Growth Factor I Levels By Octreotide In Colorectal Cancer Patients," *Gastroenterology*, Vol. 113, September 1997, pp. 767-72, PubMed, PMID:9287967.

28. Chan, June M., and Meir J. Stampfer, Edward Giovannucci, Peter H. Gann, Jing Ma, Peter Wilkinson, Charles H. Hennekens and Michael Pollak, "Plasma Insulin-like Growth factor I and Prostate Cancer risk: a prospective study," *Science*, Vol. 279, January 23, 1998, 563-66.

29. Higginbotham, Susan and Zuo-Feng Zhang, I-Min Lee, Nancy R. Cook, Edward Giovannucci, Julie E. Buring, Simin Liu, "Dietary Glycemic Load and Risk of Colorectal Cancer in the Women's Health Study," *Journal of the National Cancer Institute*, (2004) 96(3): 229-233 doi:10.1093/jnci/djh020.

30. Liu, Haibo, and Danshan Huang, David L. McArthur, Laszlo G. Boros, Nicholas Nissen, Anthony P. Heaney, "Fructose Induces Transketolase Flux to Promote Pancreatic Cancer Growth," *Cancer Research*, July 20, 2010.

31. Nothlings, Ute and Lynne R. Wilkens, Suzanne P. Murphy, Jean H. Hankin, Brian E. Henderson and Laurence N. Kolonel, "Meat and Fat Intake as Risk Factors for Pancreatic Cancer," *Journal of the National Cancer Institute*, October 5, 2005, 97 (19): 1458-1465. doi: 10.1093/jnci/dji292.

32. "Aspartame and Breast and Other Cancers," *The Western Journal of Medicine*, 1999 Nov-Dec;171(5-6):300-1.

33. Assessment of Chlorinated Pesticides and Polychlorinated Biphenyls in Adipose Breast Tissue Using a Supercritical Fluid Extraction Method. *Carcinogenesis*, 1994 Nov;15(11):2581-5.

34. "Unlabeled Milk From Cows Treated With Biosynthetic Growth Hormones: A Case Of Regulatory Abdication," *International Journal of Health Services* 1996;26(1):173-85.

35. "Organo Chlorines and breast cancer Risk by Receptor Status, Tumor Size, and Grade," (Canada). *Cancer Causes and Control.* 2001 Jun;12(5):395-404.

36. "Estrogenic Potential of Certain Pyrethroid Compounds in The Mcf-7 Human Breast Carcinoma Cell Line," *Environmental Health Perspectives.* 1999 Mar;107(3):173-7.

37. "Polychlorinated Biphenyls: Persistent Pollutants with Immunological, Neurological, and Endocrinological Consequences," *Alternative Medicine Review* 2011 Mar;16(1):5-13.

38. Gutierrez, David, "Soy Industry Promotes Health Myths to Sell More Soy Products, Says Author," *Natural News*, March 24, 2008, http://www.aturalnews.com/022882.html.

39. GreenMedInfo.com, "Biomedical Research On Genistein's Value In 140 Health Conditions," http://www.greenmedinfo.com/substance/genistein

40. "Diet and Cancer-Acrylamide, Artificial Sweeteners, Green Tea, Soy, Tomatoes and Vitamin Supplements," *Cancer Research UK*, updated September 25, 2009, http://info.cancerresearchuk.org/healthyliving/dietandhealthyeating/foodcontroversies/diet-and-cancer-acrylamide-artificial-sweeteners-green-tea-soy-tomatoes-and-vitamin-supplements.

41. Amarù, Danielle L. and Patricia D. Biondo, Catherine J. Field, "The Role of Conjugated Linoleic Acid in breast cancer Growth and Development," *The Open Nutraceuticals Journal*, 2010, 3, 30-46, http://www.benthamscience.com/open/tonutraj/articles/V003/SI0017TONUTRAJ/30TONUTRAJ.pdf.

42. Aro, A. and P. Bougnoux, F. Lavillonniere, E. Riboli, "Inverse Relation Between CLA in Adipose Breast Tissue and Risk of Breast Cancer. A Case-control Study in France," *Inform*, 10;5:S43, 1999.

43. Thompson, Lilian U. and Jian Min Chen, Tong Li, Kathrin Strasser-Weippl, Paul E. Goss, "Dietary Flaxseed Alters Tumor Biological Markers in Postmenopausal Breast Cancer," *Clinical Cancer Research*, May 16, 2005, 11; 3828, doi: 10.1158/1078-0432.CCR-04-2326.

44. Demark-Wahnefried, Wendy and Thomas J. Polascik, Stephen L. George, Boyd R. Switzer, John F. Madden, Mack T. Ruffin IV, Denise C. Snyder, Kouros Owzar, Vera Hars, David M. Albala, Philip J. Walther, Cary N. Robertson, Judd W. Moul, Barbara K. Dunn, Dean Brenner, Lori Minasian, Philip Stella, Robin T. Vollmer, "Flaxseed Supplementation (Not Dietary Fat Restriction) Reduces Prostate Cancer

Proliferation Rates in Men Presurgery," *Cancer Epidemiology, Biomarkers & Prevention*, December 2008, 17; 3577, doi: 10.1158/1055-9965.EPI-08-0008.

45. "Vitamin D and Prevention of Breast Cancer: Pooled Analysis," *The Journal of Steroid Biochemistry and Molecular Biology*, 2007 Mar;103(3-5):708-11

46. "Vitamin D Council, Vitamin D Needs": http://www.vitamindcouncil.org/about-vitamin-d/how-to-get-your-vitamin-d/vitamin-d-supplementation/

47. "Does Bodyweight Affect Cancer Risk?" American Cancer Society, last revised January 13, 2012, http://www.cancer.org/Cancer/CancerCauses/DietandPhysicalActivity/BodyWeightandCancerRisk/body-weight-and-cancer-risk-effects.

48. Holmes, Michelle D. and Wendy Y. Chen, Diane Feskanich and Graham A. Colditz, "Physical activity and survival after breast cancer diagnosis," (paper presented at the Annual Meeting of the American Association for Cancer Research in Orlando, Mar 29, 2004).

49. Cottreau, Carrie M. and Roberta B. Ness, Andrea M. Kriska, "Physical Activity and Reduced Risk of Ovarian Cancer," *Obstetrics and Gynecology*, October 2000, Volume 96, Issue 4, 609-614, http://journals.lww.com/greenjournal/Fulltext/2000/10000/Physical_Activity_and_Reduced_Risk_of_Ovarian.24. aspx.

50. "More Evidence That Exercise Prevents Cancer," PreventDisease.com, accessed June 22, 2012, http://preventdisease.com/home/tips42.shtml.

51. "Physical Activity and Cancer," *National Cancer Institute*, last reviewed July 22, 2009, http://www.cancer.gov/cancertopics/factsheet/prevention/ physicalactivity.

52. International Agency for Research on Cancer, Weight Control and Physical Activity, IARC *Handbooks of Cancer Prevention* Vol. 6, 2002, http://www.iarc. fr/en/publications/pdfs-online/prev/handbook6.

53. Ballard-Barbash, R. and C. Friedenreich, M. Slattery, L. Thune, "Obesity and Body Composition," in *Cancer Epidemiology and Prevention*, ed. D. Schottenfeld and J. F. Fraumeni, 3rd ed. (New York: Oxford University Press, 2006).

54. Lee, I. and Y. Oguma, "Physical Activity," in *Cancer Epidemiology and Prevention*, ed. D. Schottenfeld and J. F. Fraumeni, 3rd ed. (New York: Oxford University Press, 2006).

55. McTiernan, A., ed., "Cancer Prevention and Management Through Exercise and Weight Control," (Boca Raton: Taylor & Francis Group, LLC, 2006).

56. Kubik A and P. Zatloukal, L. Tomasek, J. Dolezal, L. Syllabova, J. Kara, P. Kopecky, I. Plesko, "A Case-control Study of Lifestyle and Lung Cancer Associations by Histological Types," *Neoplasma*. 2008, 55(3):192-99, PubMed, PMID: 18348651.

57. Blanchard, Christopher M. and Kerry S. Courneya, Kevin Stein, "Cancer Survivors' Adherence to Lifestyle Behavior Recommendations and Associations with Health-related Quality of Life: Results from the American Cancer Society's SCS-II," *Journal of Clinical Oncology*, May 1, 2008, 26(13):2198-204, doi: 10.1200/JCO.2007.14.6217

58. Pauk, Norbert and Antonin Kubik, Petr Zatloukal, PhD; Ladislav Tomasek, PhD; Libor Havel, MD and Jiri Dolezal, "Importance of Smoking, Diet, and Physical Exercise for the Risk of Lung Cancer in Women," *Chest*, October 2010, 138:252A, doi: 10.1378/chest.9365.

59. Forman, Michele and Carol Etzel, Somdat Mahabir, Qiong Dong, Stephanie Barrera and Margaret Spitz, "Diet and Physical Activity In Lung Cancer Risk Prediction For Current, Former, and Never Smokers," 2007, AACR Meeting Abstracts Online, http://www.aacrmeetingabstracts.org/cgi/content/meeting_abstract/2007/6_Cancer_Prevention_Meeting/B143.

60. Pinto, Bernardine M. and Georita M. Frierson, Carolyn Rabin, Joseph J. Tunzo, Bess H. Marcus, "Home-Based Physical Activity Intervention For breast cancer Patients," *Journal of Clinical Oncology*, May 20, 2005; 23(15): 3577–3587, doi: 10.1200/JCO.2005.03.080.

61. Meyerhardt, Jeffrey A. and Edward L. Giovannucci, Michelle D. Holmes, Andrew T. Chan, Jennifer A. Chan, Graham A. Colditz, Charles S. Fuchs, "Physical Activity And Survival After Colorectal Cancer Diagnosis," *Journal of Clinical Oncology*, August 1, 2006; 24(22):3527–3534, doi: 10.1200/ JCO.2006.06.0855.

62. Villanueva, Cristina M. and Kenneth P. Cantor, Will D. King, Jouni J.K. Jaakkola, Sylvaine Cordier, Charles F. Lynch, Stefano Porru, Manolis Kogevinas, "Total and Specific Fluid Consumption As Determinants Of Bladder Cancer Risk," *International Journal of Cancer*, April 15, 2006, 118(8):2040-47, DOI: 10.1002/ijc.21587.

63. Henner, Marilu and Laura Morton, The 30-Day Total Health Makeover (New York: HarperCollins, 1999).

64. "Role of Glutathione in cancer pathophysiology and therapeutic interventions." *J Exp Ther Oncol.* 2012;9(4):303-16.

65. Flavor characteristics of Glutathione in raw and cooked foodstuffs. *Biosci Biotechnol Biochem.* 1997 Dec;61(12):1977-80.

66. Rubenstein, Lori, "Forgiveness: A Healthy Alternative," *Ezine Articles*, accessed June 22, 2012, http://ezinearticles.com/?Forgiveness:-A-Healthy-Alternative&id=7088474.

67. "Secrets of A Cancer Virus Is Revealed," Press Release, Cancer Research UK, July 21, 2003, http://info.cancerresearchuk.org/news/archive/ pressrelease/2003-07-21-secrets-of-a-cancer-virus-revealed.

68. DiMasi, Joseph A. and Ronald W. Hansen, Henry G. Grabowski, "The Price of Innovation: New Estimates Of Drug Development Costs," *Journal of Health Economics*, 22 (2003) 151–185, http://www.cptech.org/ip/health/econ/dimasi2003.pdf.

69. "Quercetin," GreenMedInfo.com, accessed June 24, 2012, http://www.greenmedinfo.com/substance/quercetin.

70. Chen, H. and B. Sun, S. Wang, S. Pan, Y. Gao, X. Bai, D. Xue, "Growth Inhibitory Effects of Dihydroartemisinin on Pancreatic Cancer Cells," *Journal of Cancer Research and Clinical Oncology*, June 2010, 136(6):897-903, PubMed, PMID:19941148, http://www.ncbi.nlm.nih.gov/pubmed/19941148.

71. "Green Tea News," *Live in the Now*, accessed June 22, 2012, http://www.liveinthenow.com/news/green-tea.

72. Ichim, Thomas E. and Boris Minev, Todd Braciak, Brandon Luna, Ron Hunninghake, Nina A Mikirova, James A Jackson, Michael J Gonzalez, Jorge R Miranda-Massari, Doru T Alexandrescu, Constantin A Dasanu, Vladimir Bogin, Janis Ancans, R Brian Stevens, Boris Markosian, James Koropatnick, Chien-Shing Chen, and Neil H Riordan, "Intravenous Ascorbic Acid to Prevent and Treat Cancer-associated Sepsis?" *Journal of Translational Medicine*, March 4, 2011, DOI 10.1186/1479-5876-9-25.

73. "Intravenous Vitamin C as Cancer Therapy," Orthomolecular News Service, April 14, 2011, http://orthomolecular.org/resources/omns/v07n03.shtml.

74. Hunnington, Ron, "Intravenous Vitamin C and Cancer," (Presentation at the Medical Sciences Campus, University of Puerto Rico, April 12, 2010).

75. "Beta-Glucan," GreenMedInfo.com, accessed June 23, 2012, http://www.greenmedinfo.com/substance/Beta-Glucan.

76. Shamsuddin, A.M., "Inositol Phosphates Have Novel Anticancer Function," *Journal of Nutrition*, March 1995, 125(3 Suppl):725S-732S, PubMed, PMID: 7884558.

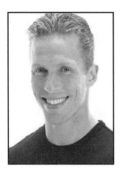

DR. BEN LERNER is the Co-founder of Maximized Living, Maximized Living Health Centers, and the Maximized Living Foundation. He owned and operated five clinics in Central Florida. These clinics cared for over 12,000 each month with a combination of pediatric, wellness care, corrective care, sports performance, personal injury, and a special attention to chronic illness.

Dr. Lerner is currently the co-chairman for the Wellness Advisory Council for sports that provides care for many of the U.S. sports governing bodies as well as with teams and athletes at the professional, college, and high school level.

He is the author of nine books and has spent multiple weeks on the *New York Times*, *Wall Street Journal*, and *USA Today* Best Sellers lists. He lives in Celebration Florida with his wife Dr. Sheri Lerner and their three children, Skylar, Nicole, and Cael.

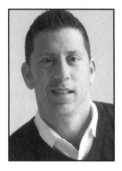

DR. CHARLES MAJORS is the co-author of two books, *Maximized Living Makeover* and *Cruise Ship or Nursing Home*. He graduated from University of Illinois with a bachelors of Science and went on to receive his doctorate degree from Palmer College of Chiropractic. He is a highly sought after speaker and has given hundreds of live lecture events in the past ten years, during which time he opened up five clinics.

In September 2010 he was diagnosed with an incurable bone marrow cancer that metastasized to his brain. He chose to leave conventional medicine and applied the same principles he had been teaching for years to reverse his own cancer and not only survive but thrive. He lives in Plainfield, Illinois, a suburb of Chicago, with his beautiful wife Andrea and their four children.

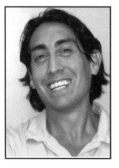

SAYER JI is the founder and editor-in-chief of GreenMedInfo. com, the world's largest, open access, evidence-based natural medicine database. His writings and research are regularly featured on thousands of websites, and have been published in a variety of journals, including *The Wellbeing Journal*, *The Journal of Gluten Sensitivity*. He is the author of *The Dark Side of Wheat*, and lectures regularly on health and wellness topics throughout the country.